THE
PICKLE JAR

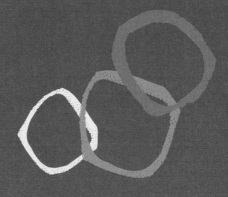

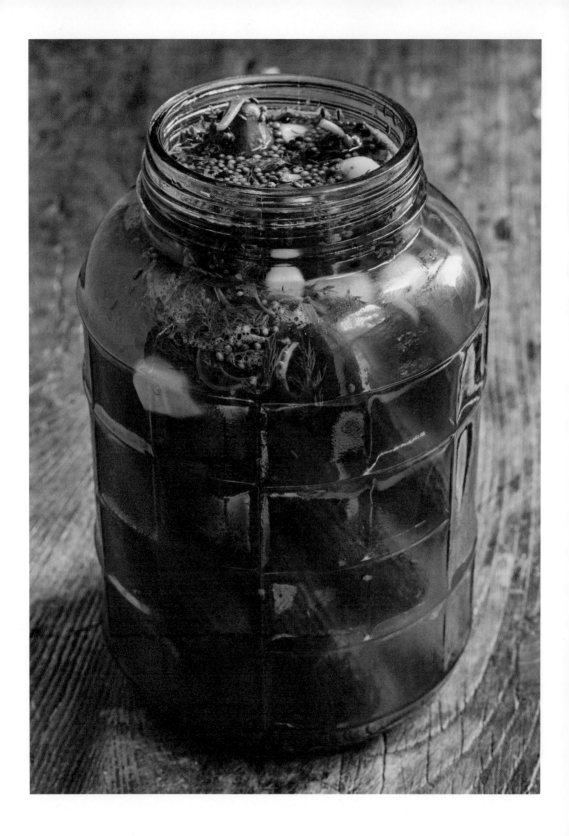

THE PICKLE JAR

Recipes for Making and Using Pickles and Ferments

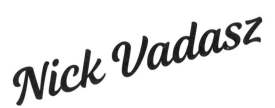

hamlyn

For Rina, whose endless love, strength and support
keeps our pickle boat afloat.

First published in Great Britain in 2025 by Hamlyn, an imprint of
Octopus Publishing Group Ltd
Carmelite House
50 Victoria Embankment
London EC4Y 0DZ
www.octopusbooks.co.uk

An Hachette UK Company
www.hachette.co.uk

Text copyright © Nick Vadasz 2025
Photography, design & layout copyright © Octopus Publishing Group 2024

Distributed in the US by Hachette Book Group
1290 Avenue of the Americas
4th and 5th Floors
New York, NY 10104

Distributed in Canada by Canadian Manda Group
664 Annette St., Toronto, Ontario, Canada M6S 2C8

ISBN 978 1 80419 274 0

A CIP catalogue record for this book is available from the British Library.

Printed and bound in China.

10 9 8 7 6 5 4 3 2 1

Commissioning Editor: Isabel Jessop
Senior Managing Editor: Sybella Stephens
Copy Editor: Lucy Bannell
Art Director & Designer: Juliette Norsworthy
Photographer: Joe Woodhouse
Food Stylist: Rosie Ramsden
Props Stylist: Florence Blair
Illustrator: Ikon Design
Production Manager: Caroline Alberti

CONTENTS

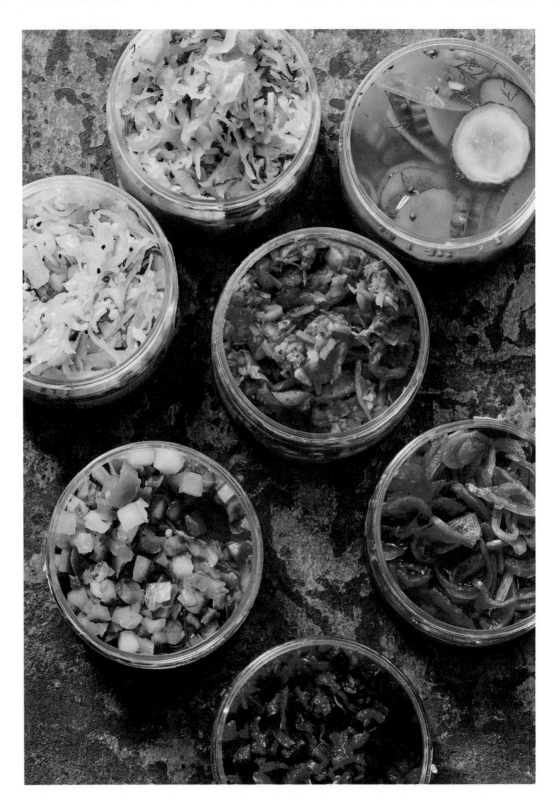

FOREWORD
by Matthew McAuliffe

Head of Inspiration and New Products at Compleat Food Group, and the guy who discovered Vadasz and provided the key to unlock the pickle dream.

Discovering exceptional products often happens unexpectedly, in the midst of everyday routine tasks or ordinary moments. For me, the journey into the world of Vadasz began amid the bustle of judging the Great Taste Awards. It was there, among a sea of flavours and aromas, that I first encountered their bread and butter pickle — since transformed into the enticing Garlic & Dill Fresh Pickles. Despite the blind tastings which are a key element of the judging process, the allure of these pickles was undeniable. Intrigued, I set out to find the source, which led me to a humble kitchen adorned with Vadasz-branded jars.
From that moment on, I was hooked.

As a regular patron of the pickle pioneer's market stalls on Venn Street in Clapham, southwest London, and the bustling Brockley Market in Lewisham, southeast London, I witnessed first-hand the dedication and passion that fuelled Nick's craft. It was only a matter of time before the opportunity arose to collaborate and bring Vadasz pickles to a wider audience via the counters of supermarket delis.

My journey with Vadasz was one of immersion into the art, science and magic of fermentation under the guidance of Nick, the mastermind behind these delectable creations. Together with an exceptional team, we delved into the fundamentals and mysteries of lacto-fermentation, eventually culminating in the successful launch of Vadasz pickles and ferments, now found in the aisles of almost every British supermarket.

From naturally fermented Garlic & Dill Sauerkraut and vibrant Super-Beet Kimchi to cold-brined Red Onion Fresh Pickles, Vadasz offers condiments that are guaranteed to make every meal even more delicious. And now, with the publication of this book, Nick invites you into his magical realm, where pickles and ferments are not just condiments, but transformative ingredients.

I am thrilled to see Nick's imagination, expertise and passion captured within these pages, offering practical advice on everything from kick-starting your own kimchi to perfecting your pickle. It is a testament to the belief that pickling and fermenting aren't just processes — they're a way of life, a journey of exploration and discovery.

So, as you embark on your own culinary adventure, armed with Nick's wisdom about the magic of brining and fermentation, I invite you to savour every moment. For here you will find not only recipes but illuminating stories — stories of tradition, culture, innovation and the timeless joy of good food.

INTRODUCTION
by Nick Vadasz

Back in 1956, at the time of the Hungarian Revolution, when the Soviet Union
invaded Hungary to crush the uprising, my grandmother left the country with
my father, and she left in a hurry. They had to leave most things behind and
just grabbed what they could — the important stuff: a few pieces of family silver,
a bunch of old photos, a suitcase full of clothes and…a big jar of pickles.
Why the pickles? Well, as Gran said, *'We didn't know when we were going
to eat again, so pickles seemed like a good idea!'*
Those pickles turned out to be a great idea, Gran… To this day, we always
have Gran's pickles (not the original ones, of course!) with every meal, and all
these years later, our family still keeps an extra-big jar in the fridge for Gran.
Just in case.

MY DAD TAUGHT ME TO COOK

*'Salt the cucumbers for longer and they'll be
crunchier.'*
'Add more sugar, it's too sour!'
'Not too much garlic!'

There he goes again, reminding me what
I should be doing with the *uborka saláta*
(fresh cucumber pickle).

No point reminding him that I'm now The
Picklesman and that we have a big pickle
brand with his name on it too! Of course,
he's right — you never ever stop learning.
Dad never actually taught me to cook. It was
more like I was a fully engaged, passionate
observer, and this facilitated my learning.

When he cooked, I absorbed the smells, flavours and
the rituals around familiar meals, such as chicken
paprika, chicken schnitzel or, our absolute favourite,
stuffed peppers. Understanding the methodologies
and recipes soon followed. Sometimes helping, for
example forming meatballs and then using them to
stuff the green peppers, and watching him make
things like the roux for the sweet tomato sauce that
the peppers cooked in, meant that cooking slowly
became part of me. I absorbed knowledge in the
same way as the meatballs, flecked with grains
of rice and simple seasonings, absorbed the rich,
sweet, paprika-spiced tomato sauce they bathed in.
I wallowed in this bath of culinary knowledge, happy
as a pig in mud!

Cooking with Dad became a routine I loved and
looked forward to, never boring or tedious but always
entertaining and fun.

I was, of course, always incentivized by the reward:
the most delicious Hungarian food.

I still cook with my dad. We recently had a big family
gathering for Easter, and Dad, less active but still
totally involved and at the helm, steered me from
his chair in the kitchen, offering familiar advice and
anecdotes from a full life in the kitchen.

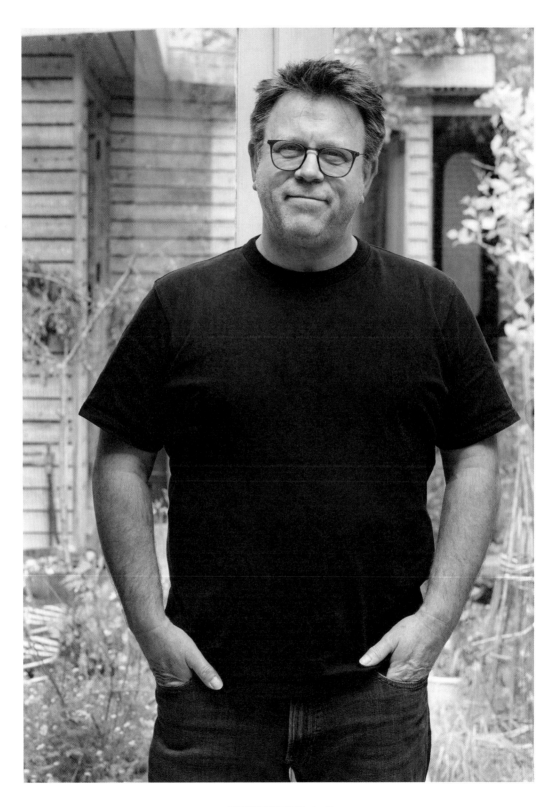

A LOVE OF PICKLES

As a child growing up in the UK, a pickle was mostly a challenging way to eat vegetables – extremely sour and often tasting only of strong onion and the brining. Luckily, there were some good Eastern European brands that transitioned my palate and helped to ease me into their crunchy, sour and sweet pleasures.

But the pickles I really enjoyed, the ones I grew to love, were those prepared by my Hungarian grandmother and dad: peeled, freshly sliced cucumbers salted for a while, then rinsed, squeezed until no liquid remained and submerged in a brine of vinegar, water, garlic and sugar. There they sat for just an hour or less and absorbed the acidic, sweet, garlicky brine in which they bathed.

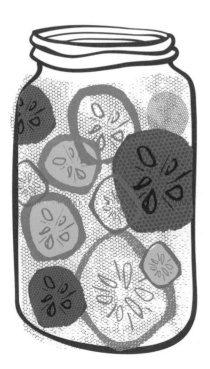

When lunch or dinner was served, the *uborka saláta* appeared at the table, piled high like a mountain in a small bowl, adorned with a flash of white soured cream and a big pinch of paprika; a beacon welcoming us to the table. The aroma of fresh cucumbers, reminiscent of newly mown grass in summer, together with the sharp but perfectly balanced taste of the brine that continued to develop as the meal progressed was, and still is, a joy. It's a memory of childhood that resonates through time to my table today and to my children's future tables too.

Fast forward to early adult life, when art college somehow led me to a commercial kitchen where I honed the cooking skills I'd assimilated during my childhood. A love-hate relationship followed: a love for food, the cooking process and the banter of a busy kitchen versus a hatred of chaotic, busy services and the challenges of coping under extreme pressure. How could I sustain a career in food and yet banish the crazy hours and stressful environment?

Frustrated by the antisocial hours, I left the kitchen work when my first child was a toddler and I took up teaching English in a further education college. While making use of the long holidays, I kept some skin in the game with catering and then later on with street food. It was the street food that opened the door to the opportunity I'd been dreaming of. Soon the queues for the pickles I served became longer than those for the quesadillas they came with. I quickly became The Picklesman, making and supplying markets, delis, shops, restaurants and street food stalls across London and beyond.

Demand expanded and I soon outgrew the shipping container in Hackney, east London, where I began, and moved on to a bigger production unit where we ('we' because by then I employed local people) built and continued to grow, supplying larger customers who all needed more and more pickles and ferments.

I'd always had a vision of our pickles and ferments lined up on the shelves at supermarkets – I wanted everyone across the UK to enjoy the tastes and benefits of good-quality pickles, kimchi and sauerkraut. That vision became reality when Matt McAuliffe knocked on my arch door in 2017 and asked if Vadasz would be interested in appearing alongside several carefully curated food makers in a pop-up deli — 'Umm, yes please!' was my response. This gave us the opportunity we needed to prove demand was there, and persuade Matt and his colleagues to get Vadasz on board. After a few years of hard graft and development, the transition was complete: Vadasz became a member of The Compleat Food Group family and are now on the shelves of the UK's favourite retailers.

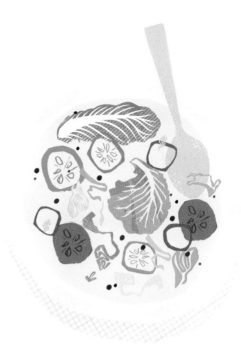

A PICKLE REVOLUTION OR EVOLUTION?

Nowadays, walk into a decent restaurant and you will probably see a side of house pickles offered on the menu. Kimchi's popularity is so high that it appears not only in Korean restaurants, but across menus in many different forms. Kimchi is king: versatile, tangy, spicy and umami, it's also packed with healthy ingredients.

So why are we all getting hooked on pickles and ferments? People of my grandmother's generation and those preceding it were raised eating fermented foods. They had a varied yet natural diet, where farm-to-table eating wasn't just a 21st-century lifestyle choice but a way of life. The only food processing came through making cheeses, sausages, charcuterie, wines and beers. And as was the case with vegetables too, this often involved fermentation as a method of preservation. These staples were traditionally made at the end of the summer growing season, utilizing the forthcoming low winter temperatures to aid the process. The gradual change to industrialized farming, growing and manufacturing throughout the 20th century saw a move away from simple, seasonal community food traditions. This was consolidated post-war as more people, both men and women, began to work and spend less time at home, meaning less time for old food-making traditions and an increasing demand for convenience foods.

However, the beginning of the 21st century saw a new generation of people hungry for old knowledge and nostalgic for ancient traditions and practices.

Soon after I began selling pickles on market stalls across London, I was inundated with requests for workshops. This new breed of foodies was driven by a desire to understand the methods and magic of fermentation. Some were fascinated by the science and the developing evidence around the health benefits, while others were impressed by the taste and the versatility of ferments. Drawing on my lived experience and the knowledge I'd gained over the years, I was able to give people an opportunity to learn the preserving traditions that we have lost over time.

A renaissance, a revival, an evolution, but not a revolution. In fact, I'm very proud that, like the generations before, we make ferments the old-fashioned way: simply and naturally. The interest in and popularity of fermented vegetables such as kimchi, sauerkraut and pickles, keeps growing year on year, fuelled by a commitment to eat healthier and less-processed foods that taste amazing and add true value to whatever it is you're making.

A HEALTHY GUT

By eating fermented vegetables, you are helping to maintain a balance of 'friendly' lactic acid bacteria (LAB) in your gut – which exist in their billions in raw, unpasteurized, fermented kimchi and sauerkraut – and can enjoy multiple health benefits (see opposite).

The key to promoting a healthy gut is to incorporate fermented vegetables and pickles into your meals as part of a diverse and varied diet, thereby putting plants, beneficial bacteria, extra nutrients and fibre centre stage.

In this book you will discover how to use and get the most out of your pickles and ferments at every meal of the day.

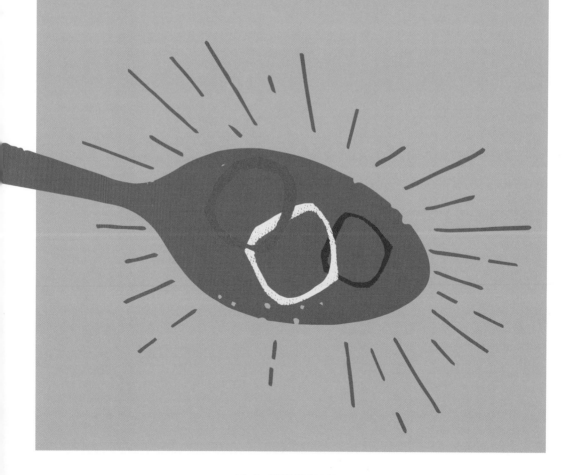

THE HEALTH BENEFITS OF FERMENTED VEGETABLES

By Dr Sarah Schenker, registered dietitian and nutritionist

IMPROVES DIGESTIVE HEALTH. Fermented vegetables contain probiotics that can help to restore the balance of the gut microbiome (the 'friendly' bacteria in the gut). They also provide prebiotic fibres that are a nourishing food source for the probiotic bacteria, which in turn boosts their number.

FOOD IS EASIER TO DIGEST. Fermentation breaks down nutrients in foods, which makes them easier to digest

BOOSTS IMMUNITY. Fermented vegetables increase the diversity of the gut microbiome, which is associated with improved immune function. Probiotic bacteria can help to mobilize immune cells and enhance the body's defence against infections and diseases.

REDUCES SYMPTOMS OF STRESS AND ANXIETY. Chronic high levels of the hormone cortisol can cause inflammation, which is associated with stress and anxiety. A healthy gut microbiome reduces inflammation and can help to control cortisol levels.

REDUCES RISK OF DEPRESSION. Gut function and mental health are closely linked by the gut-brain axis. Fermented vegetables improve the gut microbiome and have a positive influence on mental health.

REDUCES RISK OF CANCER. Probiotic bacteria produce sphingolipids, which have anticarcinogenic effects.

AIDS WEIGHT LOSS. Probiotic bacteria produce short chain fatty acids, which can help to improve satiety — the feeling of being full.

REDUCES RISK OF DIABETES AND METABOLIC SYNDROME. Fermented vegetables are associated with reducing inflammatory substances, which are linked to diabetes.

LOWERS CHOLESTEROL LEVELS. The short chain fatty acids produced by probiotic bacteria prevent excessive production of cholesterol, while increased bacterial activity in the gut enhances bile acid deconjugation, positively affecting cholesterol metabolism.

LOWERS BLOOD PRESSURE. Fermented vegetables contain nitrites that can help to lower blood pressure, while probiotic bacteria produce conjugated linoleic acids, which also have blood pressure-lowering effects.

INCREASES ANTIOXIDANT ACTIVITY. The process of fermentation breaks down antioxidant substances in vegetables, making them more bioavailable.

REDUCTION OF ANTI-NUTRITIONAL COMPOUNDS. The process of fermentation can reduce the concentration of anti-nutritional compounds found in vegetables, such as phytic acids, which can bind to nutrients and stop them being absorbed in the body.

See pages 156–7 for references and further reading.

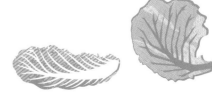

WHAT IS A PICKLE?

A pickle is an acidified vegetable. That's it? Well no, because dairy, meat and fish can also be pickled, but they all go through a process that involves acidification one way or another. I tend to stick to pickling veggies or the occasional egg, so in this book we will focus mainly on vegetable pickles, plus a little fruit.

THE TWO PICKLE TYPES

There are two main types of pickle: one where you add acid to vegetables to preserve them, and the other (clever ones) where the vegetables ferment in their own preserving acid.

1

VINEGAR BRINING is where acid, usually vinegar, is used to preserve vegetables. The vinegar prevents the growth of bacteria, yeasts and pathogens, resulting in a safe environment where salt, spices/aromatics, herbs and often sugar are added to create flavourful brines that, as well as preserving, give flavour to the vegetables submerged in them.

Vadasz vinegar pickles are cold-brined, meaning that the brine is not heated prior to submerging the vegetables. This protects the flavour, texture and nutrients of the resulting pickles. Our pickles are never pasteurized or heat-treated either.

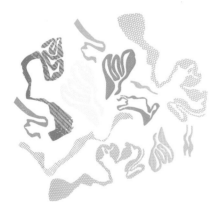

2

FERMENTATION is when salt is added to water to create a brine in which whole vegetables are fermented, or salt is added to sliced or shredded vegetables to create sauerkraut or kimchi. The vegetables are submerged in their brine and covered to create an anaerobic (oxygen-free/airtight) environment in which to ferment — an essential part of lactic acid bacteria (LAB) fermentation.

When making kimchi or sauerkraut, the cut or shredded vegetables are mixed with salt. As a consequence, water is drawn out of the vegetables and this water becomes brine. Within the brine, beneficial microbes/LAB grow and produce lactic acid, which in turn preserves the vegetables and gives the familiar sour tang.

As the vegetables are left to ferment over a few days — or even weeks, depending on the temperature of the environment — they will change and develop. It's a dynamic process where you, the maker, are the custodian of the product, but it will essentially make itself. Or, to be more accurate, it will develop in texture, flavour and acidity on its own, with your only input being the preparation and then deciding when to stop or slow down the fermentation process by refrigerating it — or eating it!

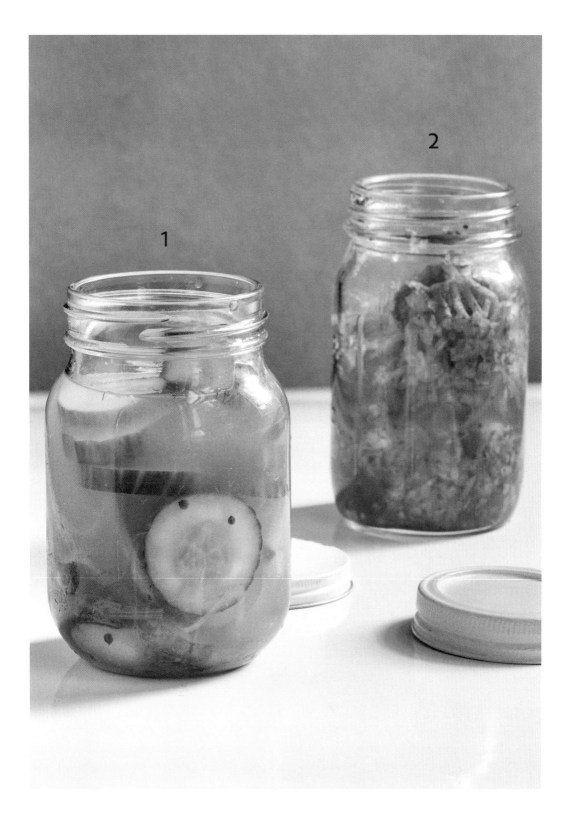

FRESH VERSUS AMBIENT

'Nick, I went looking for your pickles and couldn't find them. Why?'
'Our pickles are chilled. Did you check the chilled deli aisle
— you know, near the hummus?' I repeat frequently.

Walk into any supermarket, locate the condiments aisle and you will be
confronted with a wall of jars. From mayo, mustard and horseradish to
pickles, relishes, ketchups and hot sauces, you'll even find sauerkraut
and kimchi there too. But no Vadasz. This is because Vadasz pickles
and ferments are all made fresh and never pasteurized or heat-treated,
so they must be kept chilled. There are two main reasons why we don't
follow the processes of all those products on the ambient aisles:

★ To achieve the best-tasting product possible, all our pickles are
   sliced, cold-brined in vinegar, and seasoned with herbs and spices
   before being refrigerated, retaining all the goodness of the fresh
   vegetables, with a more complex yet fresher, cleaner taste than those
   pickles that are pasteurized. In other words, we don't cook all that
   flavour out.

★ To retain the 'friendly' gut bacteria and its benefits, all our ferments,
   such as sauerkraut and kimchi, are lacto-fermented using traditional
   methods, which help to preserve the vegetables without the need
   to pasteurize. And, of course, just like the cold-brined pickles, raw,
   naturally fermented and unpasteurized also means better, richer and
   more complex flavours too.

So when you're next in your local supermarket and you stroll past the wall
of ambient condiments and see kimchi or sauerkraut, remember: if it's
ambient, it's not chilled; if it's not chilled, then it's been pasteurised;
if it's pasteurized, all the good stuff — that healthy gut-promoting bacteria
— has been killed off.

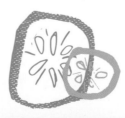

IT'S FERMENT TO BE

The trouble with getting people on board with fermentation is the association we make with things that we shouldn't eat. Negative phrases come to mind: 'It's gone off', 'It's gone bad', 'It's gone fizzy' and so on.

The way we interpret food varies depending on our experience, cultural food heritage and the context. What we perceive as 'good' or 'bad' is subjective and dependent on the rules by which we have been bought up or our lived experience.

My Hungarian grandmother would place a half bottle of milk on the windowsill in the summer for the sun to warm and ferment it over several days before gulping it down, enjoying the sour tang and perhaps knowing it had health-giving qualities too – she lived to 93 years old. Although I didn't take to drinking it back then, the fact that this lived experience, this formative knowledge, was instilled in me from an early age surely made me more likely to embrace the yogurt, kefir and ayran that I grew to love later.

We often forget that the tanginess, sourness and often funkiness we get through fermentation are characteristics common in very familiar, everyday foods and drinks, such as real ales and ciders, Stilton or mature Cheddar cheese, and Worcestershire, Tabasco and soy sauces.

So it's not such a stretch to see why, when people try sauerkraut or kimchi a few times, it grows on them rapidly. The sensory joy of fermented vegetables, as well as their health benefits, means that their popularity is surging, and Vadasz is helping to bring them to the people. It's now more often love at first bite, so it was definitely ferment to be!

In Part One, on the following pages, there are eight traditional recipes for using fermentation as the method of pickling. Each of these can and should be adapted to create as many variations as you wish.

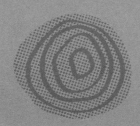

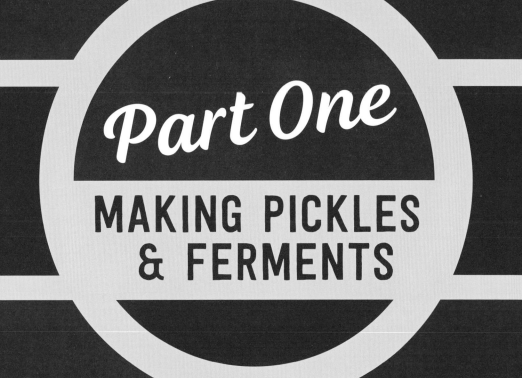

Part One

MAKING PICKLES & FERMENTS

Fermented Fruit & Veg

Here are some key techniques you will need for the fermented vegetable recipes in this chapter.

SUBMERGING YOUR FERMENTS

Your fermented vegetables need to be fully submerged in their brine to ferment efficiently, and there are a couple of different methods you can use, as follows.

WEIGHTED SECOND CONTAINER

When using a large food storage container for fermenting, such as a 4-litre (7-pint) recycled ice-cream tub, as suggested in the recipes, fill a second lidded container of the same size with water and put the lid on. Place directly on top of your fermenting vegetables so that they are compacted beneath. The quantity/weight of water may need to be adjusted during the fermentation period as the brine level in your fermenting container increases. And you may need to remove some brine from the lower container to prevent too much escaping. Don't waste the surplus — add it to a stir-fry or salad dressing.

Carefully cover the stacked containers with a muslin cloth or clean tea towel to prevent any flies or other unwanted visitors getting in.

During the fermentation process, the CO_2 gas created by the lactic acid bacteria (LAB) as they consume all the natural sugars present in the vegetables will often cause brine to seep out of the top of your container, so place the containers in a suitable vessel for the brine to overflow into.

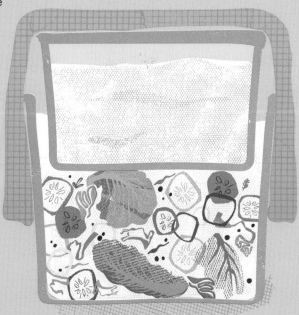

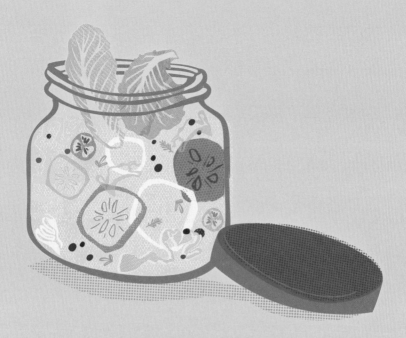

SMALLER LIDDED CONTAINER

If using smaller lidded food storage containers for fermenting, such as your used but thoroughly cleaned Vadasz pots, your brine and ingredients may already reach the top of the container once packed. In this case, simply cover with clean surplus cabbage leaves or other vegetable trimmings, or some baking paper or clingfilm so that this top layer sits proud of the top of the container. As you secure the lid, it will push the ingredients down into the brine, creating the anaerobic (oxygen-free/airtight) seal you need.

If your ingredients don't reach the top of the container once packed, place some scrunched-up unused freezer bags on top of them to fill the gap, then when you put the lid on they will push the ingredients down into the brine. Don't worry if the brine overflows, as this indicates minimal headspace at the top of the container, giving you the requisite anaerobic conditions.

As with the first method, place the containers in a suitable vessel for the brine to overflow into.

'BURPING' YOUR FERMENTS

You will need to 'burp' your fermented vegetables to release the CO_2 that builds up, by loosening the lid if using a jar or container with a closed, tight-fitting lid. This will not be necessary if using a weighted container, as the CO_2 will escape between the containers' gaps. This can be quite a frequent job in higher temperatures and depending on what you are fermenting. For example, when the natural sugars in tomatoes are coupled with garlic, the resulting fermented tomatoes will produce a lot more CO_2 than, say, celery.

FERMENTING TOP TIPS

★ **SALT QUANTITY.** Do you like to discover a new place you're visiting by wandering around, or do you prefer to follow a map without the risk of getting lost? Both approaches can get you to the same point, but I've always learned more on the journey than at the destination, albeit taking me a while longer! It's your choice and what suits your learning style best: you can weigh all your prepped ingredients to determine how much salt to add – about 2% of the total weight– or go freestyle, adding salt and mixing, then tasting until the vegetables are quite a bit saltier than you would be willing to eat. Difficult to quantify, I know, but once you've done it a few times, it will become more intuitive and, as the salting may vary the outcome slightly, more interesting too.

★ **TO PEEL OR NOT TO PEEL.** There is no need to peel root vegetables, such as carrots, daikon and beetroot. Most come pre-washed or 'clean' and it's good practice to retain the skins to allow the remaining, post-washed yeasts to feed the fermentation process.

★ **YEAST GROWTH.** In warmer weather, if you are attempting to ferment beyond 2 weeks, you may get small amounts of white yeast growth, commonly manifesting as a white film on top of the kimchi or the surface of the brine. This is harmless and can be removed easily, and what's beneath should be fine. But it does indicate that the kimchi or the briny surface has become oxidized (exposed to air), so once you have discarded the top 1–2cm (½–¾ inch), you should cover thoroughly to minimize the exposure to air and therefore mitigate the risk of further yeast growth.

★ **TEMPERATURE AND TIME.** I have eaten kimchi that I've fermented for 2–3 months at low temperatures and eaten batches over a year old, some really funky, some really fresh. Experimenting with temperatures and timings is fun and can result in rewarding deep flavours and textures, but remember that the best tools to judge the quality of your ferments are your palate, nose and eyes, and over time of course your experience will guide your approach more and more.

★ **ANAEROBIC FERMENTATION.** Although anaerobic fermentation (without oxygen/air) often ensures the best results for kimchi making, it isn't always necessary and you shouldn't be too concerned about this aspect of the process unless you are fermenting vegetables over a long period of time or in large quantities. Here I have given the best method to avoid any problems, but most homemade kimchi or sauerkraut will ferment within 1–2 weeks, so yeast growth – and its potential for spoilage – will be minimal in any case.

★ **FERMENTING FRUIT.** Fermenting fruit successfully is a tricky business because of all the natural sugars it contains. These sugars are what lactic acid bacteria (LAB) need to be able to thrive and grow, and in turn produce an acidic brine for preserving. The salt helps to leach those sugars out, but also inhibits the growth of spoiling yeasts and bacteria to some degree, depending on the quantity used. Fruits that are particularly high in natural sugars, such as mango or pineapple and strawberries (see page 36), run the risk of yeast fermentation winning out over lacto acid fermentation, resulting in an alcoholic brine and very fizzy fruit, which is not what we are after.

So how do we control the process? Increasing the salt level or adding vinegar will inhibit the growth of bacteria and yeasts. However, too much salt will prevent fermentation altogether and also render the fruit inedible unless desalinated before use. And too much vinegar will pickle rather than ferment. We need to find the sweet spot of fermenting with slightly more salt for the right amount of time and at a lower temperature. With many variables that can affect the outcome, it's wise to be cautious and try different methods as you progress. Pineapple, Strawberry & Cucumber Salsa (see page 36) is good place to start.

INTRODUCING KIMCHI

Kimchi is reputed to be among the top five healthiest foods in the world. As Korea's best-known, favourite fermented food, kimchi is embedded in Korean culture and, along with other fermented fundamentals, is the very heart and soul of Korean cuisine.

Korea has a National Kimchi Day held in November, which is considered ideal kimchi-making time before the weather gets too cold. It's when Korean families prepare big batches of kimchi to store and enjoy in the weeks and months ahead — a day to share what's been made with neighbours and friends. The recipe varies from one family to another, and that diversity is what keeps kimchi alive.

Kimchi is traditionally served with grilled meats or stir-fried with rice, but is becoming a very popular garnish, condiment and ingredient across the globe, appearing with or in everything from a cheeseburger to a burrito. In salads and sandwiches it gives an amazing hit of warm, sour chilli, garlic and ginger.

With the added nutritional value of it being raw, live and full of good bacteria, kimchi ticks all the right boxes. And, fortunately, you don't have to wait until November to make a batch. So overleaf is my recipe that, like Vadasz Kimchi, is pure, natural, vegan and free of any artificial sweeteners or thickeners.

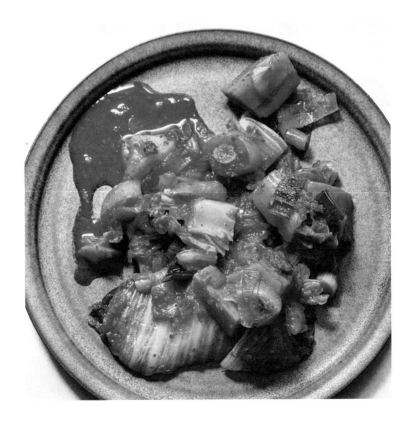

KIMCHI

2 heads of Chinese leaves, about 600–800g (1lb 5oz–1lb 12oz) each, cored, quartered lengthways and cut into big pieces

600g (1lb 5oz) mixed carrots and daikon (or any radishes or other root/hard vegetables that you can eat raw, such as turnips, celeriac or kohlrabi – even fennel and rhubarb ferment really well too), scrubbed if needed and cut into 2–4cm (¾–1½-inch) pieces

2 big bunches (about 10–12) spring onions, chopped

1 garlic bulb, cloves peeled

100g (3½oz) fresh root ginger, chopped

75g (2¾oz) gochugaru (Korean red pepper powder)

water, to blend

about 2 tablespoons fine natural sea salt

You will need 2 large lidded plastic food storage containers of the same size, each about 4 litres (7 pints) in capacity – reusing thoroughly cleaned ice-cream tubs with lids are perfect.

Wash all the vegetables thoroughly, then drain and add to a very large mixing bowl.

Put the garlic, ginger and gochugaru in a food processor or blender and blend with just enough water to form a paste.

Weigh all the vegetables and the paste then calculate 2% of that figure. Add that amount of salt or add the 2 tablespoons listed.

Add the paste and salt to the vegetables and mix well with your hands, then gently rub into the vegetables. Now try a bit – it should taste saltier than you would like to eat it (see Salt Quantity on page 22). Your veg mix should become slightly limp, and the juices drawn from the vegetables by the salt should start to appear. This liquid contains the vegetables' sugars that naturally occurring yeasts will begin to work on, creating an environment in which lactic acid bacteria (LAB) will begin to grow, and over time help to create the wonderful deep, tangy taste of fermented kimchi.

Pack the kimchi into lidded food storage containers of your choice, then submerge fully in its brine following the weighted second container method or the smaller lidded container method on page 20.

Leave to ferment at room temperature for 3–5 days, tasting every few days to check progress and to ensure the brine is covering the kimchi or at least remains as anaerobic as possible.

After 3–5 days you should have a tasty, tangy kimchi, as it ferments quickly in a warm ambient temperature. However, long, low and slow is best, so I would recommend storing it in the coolest part of your home/kitchen in summer, and somewhere slightly warmer in the winter. It may need 10 days or more in colder weather – keep tasting and leave as long as you need to achieve your desired flavour. When it's to your taste, store in the fridge as it is, or divide between smaller lidded food storage containers to keep for up to 3 months or so, but most likely you'll be eating it with everything and it won't last long!

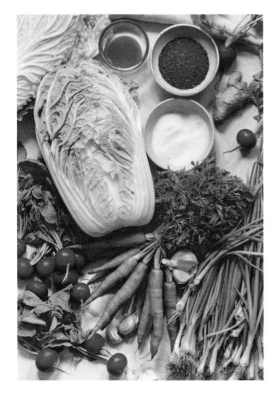

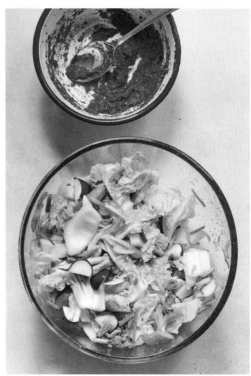

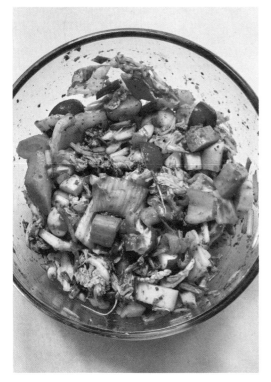

VARIATION: BEETROOT KIMCHI

As well as having a deep, earthy flavour, a gorgeous colour and many well-documented health benefits, beetroot contains good natural sugars that make it a great choice for kimchi.

To create a delicious beetroot kimchi, simply add 500g (1lb 2oz) raw, fresh beetroot (not in vinegar), scrubbed and grated or diced (or both, for texture) to the ingredients opposite and mix through, then follow the same method.

Stir through Greek yogurt seasoned with olive oil and fresh herbs, or use in recipes such as Super-Beet Kimchi Pancake with Purple Sriracha on page 55 or Carlin Peas, Cavolo Nero & Beetroot Kimchi with Dill on page 101.

SAUERKRAUT WITH GARLIC & DILL

The aim here, as with all vegetable lactic acid fermentation or lacto-fermentation as it's commonly referred to, is to create an acidic brine by shredding cabbage, adding salt along with a few spices and then mixing/rubbing/bruising the vegetable to encourage the release of its natural juices. The cabbage submerged in the brine ferments anaerobically (without oxygen/air), producing lactic acid bacteria (LAB), and this is what preserves, adds that deep sour/salty/tangy flavour and so creates the classic sauerkraut result.
Remember that the longer you leave the cabbage to ferment, the stronger the flavour will be. Taste regularly to decide when to refrigerate and therefore stop or slow down the fermentation (usually within 1–4 weeks). The ambient temperature of the room where you ferment your cabbage is a big factor in this process, and long, low and slow is a good rule of thumb for making great-tasting sauerkraut. Having said that, you can successfully make sauerkraut at the height of summer or in warm environments (20°C/68°F and above). It will just need to be refrigerated sooner than if fermented at lower temperatures.

2 whole cabbages, about 1kg (2lb 4oz), usually white cabbage but red or green cabbage, such as hispi/sweetheart, January King or Savoy, can all make good sauerkraut

20g (¾oz) fine natural sea salt, or 2% of the total weight of the other ingredients

3 garlic cloves, crushed

1 handful of dill, chopped

4 fresh bay leaves

2 teaspoons caraway seeds

2 teaspoons black peppercorns

1 teaspoon crushed juniper berries

Carefully halve the cabbages and remove the base of the core by making a V-shaped cut. Also remove any dirty or bruised outer leaves. Wash the cabbages thoroughly and drain.

Shred the cabbages using a mandoline or a food processor fitted with a slicing attachment, then place in the largest mixing bowl you have. Alternatively, if you think you might be making sauerkraut regularly, treat yourself to a big new washing-up bowl or similar — you need enough space not only to hold the cabbage but also to mix and massage it.

Add the salt, garlic, herbs and spices and mix really well with your hands to ensure everything is thoroughly combined and there are no salt-free patches, which could result in a poor fermentation and soft texture.

As you toss and mix, you will notice the cabbage becoming glossy and wet as the salt begins to draw out the juices from the cabbage. Once you're happy that it's well mixed, start to lean into it more as you continue to mix, bruising the cabbage with the heel of your hands and squeezing before releasing and repeating, breaking down the cells of the cabbage and allowing the salt to do its job effectively. Soon you will have some brine pooling in the bottom of your bowl.

Pack the cabbage into lidded food storage containers of your choice, then submerge your sauerkraut fully in its brine following the weighted second container method or the smaller lidded container method on page 20.

Leave to ferment at room temperature for 3–5 days, tasting every few days to check progress and to ensure the brine is covering the sauerkraut or at least remains as anaerobic as possible. You can eat it after just a few days, as it will ferment quickly in warm temperatures. However, remember that long, low and slow is best, so store in the coolest part of your house or kitchen in summer, and somewhere slightly warmer in the winter.

If using the small lidded container method, 'burp' your fermenting cabbage every 2 days, as directed on page 21.

After 3–5 days you should have a tasty, tangy sauerkraut, but you may need 10 days or more if making it in cold weather – keep tasting and leave as long as you need to achieve your desired flavour. When it's to your taste, store in the fridge as it is, or divide between smaller lidded food storage containers to keep for up to 3 months or so.

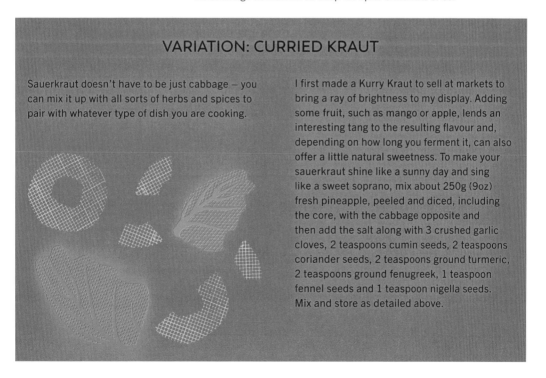

VARIATION: CURRIED KRAUT

Sauerkraut doesn't have to be just cabbage – you can mix it up with all sorts of herbs and spices to pair with whatever type of dish you are cooking.

I first made a Kurry Kraut to sell at markets to bring a ray of brightness to my display. Adding some fruit, such as mango or apple, lends an interesting tang to the resulting flavour and, depending on how long you ferment it, can also offer a little natural sweetness. To make your sauerkraut shine like a sunny day and sing like a sweet soprano, mix about 250g (9oz) fresh pineapple, peeled and diced, including the core, with the cabbage opposite and then add the salt along with 3 crushed garlic cloves, 2 teaspoons cumin seeds, 2 teaspoons coriander seeds, 2 teaspoons ground turmeric, 2 teaspoons ground fenugreek, 1 teaspoon fennel seeds and 1 teaspoon nigella seeds. Mix and store as detailed above.

FERMENTED CUCUMBER PICKLES

Generically referred to as dill pickles in the USA, in Hungarian these are called *kovászos uborka*, which translates as sourdough sun pickles or summer pickles, as they are fermented using the heel of a loaf of sourdough/rye bread stuffed into the top of the storage jar or container filled with freshly picked cucumbers, water, salt, garlic and dill. They are then left out in the heat of the summer sun to ferment, which happens very quickly (1–3 days), as the combination of high temperature and the natural yeasts in the bread activate lactic acid bacteria (LAB), which then produce the acid that turns the cucumbers into pickles. I still sometimes make these in the traditional way, weather permitting, but they are also very good made using the method below.

There are three stages or categories of these pickles, depending on the fermentation period, though the timings will vary according to the ambient temperature. These cucumber pickle variants are like those they serve at Katz's Deli in New York or those that were to be found in the Jewish delis of London's East End up until the 1980s, when most of them moved out to the suburbs.

★ **New greens** – 1–2 days may be all that's needed for these salty cucumbers, hardly fermented at all and still retaining their fresh colour.

★ **Half sours** – leave for 5–7 days for a result similar to the traditional *kovászas uborka*; mottled in colour between bright green and olive green, and somewhere between a cucumber and a pickle.

★ **Full sours** – fermented for 2–3 weeks or more, often at a lower temperature to ensure a good texture over a longer period of time. Another distinction here, and a good indication of maturity, is that the longer the ferment, the cloudier the appearance of the brine, which is a natural result of the LAB developing within it.

Serve these pickles on the side of everything, or chopped up/sliced in sandwiches and salads. In many Eastern European countries, a shot of the fermented pickle brine is drunk as a healthy tonic and reputed to be a great hangover cure too. It's also wonderful as an ingredient in cocktails and alongside vodka (or Bourbon or whisky) as a Ukrainian Pickleback (see recipe on page 154).

1.5kg (3lb 5oz) mini cucumbers

fine natural sea salt – 4% of the weight of water (e.g. 4% of 2kg/4lb 8oz water = 80g/2¾oz = salt)

1 garlic bulb, cloves separated but left unpeeled, and bruised or lightly crushed

1 tablespoon dill seeds (optional)

1 tablespoon caraway seeds

½ tablespoon coriander seeds

½ tablespoon black peppercorns

1 handful of wild fennel (if you can get it) or dill

You will need either a large jar with lid, or 2 large lidded plastic food storage containers of the same size, each about 4 litres (7 pints) in capacity – thoroughly cleaned ice-cream tubs with lids are perfect.

Wash the cucumbers well and drain.

Place the cucumbers in your container or jar and fill with fresh cold water to cover – try to ensure they all fit without leaving too much head room. Drain the water into a large mixing bowl on kitchen scales to weigh it. Add 4% of the weight of the water in salt and whisk briskly until dissolved.

Pour the brine back into the container with the cucumbers, add all the garlic and spices, and finally add the fennel or dill to the top. This should ideally be sitting proud of the container so that when you put the lid on, the ingredients will be pushed down into the brine. If not, follow the weighted second container method or the smaller lidded container method on page 20.

Place the container on a tray to catch the brine, as it may leak a bit, and leave the cucumbers to ferment in your kitchen for 2 or 3 days before checking their progress, unless you want new greens, which will need only 1–2 days in the brine.

If using the small lidded container method, 'burp' your fermenting cucumber every day, as directed on page 21.

When the pickles are to your taste, either new greens at 1–2 days or half sours at 5–7 days (see opposite), store in the fridge as they are, or divide between smaller lidded food storage containers to keep for up to 3 months or so. Their flavour will improve over time. I tend to leave some out to eat over a couple of days and put the rest in the fridge for when I need them.

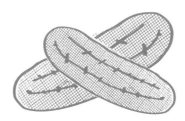

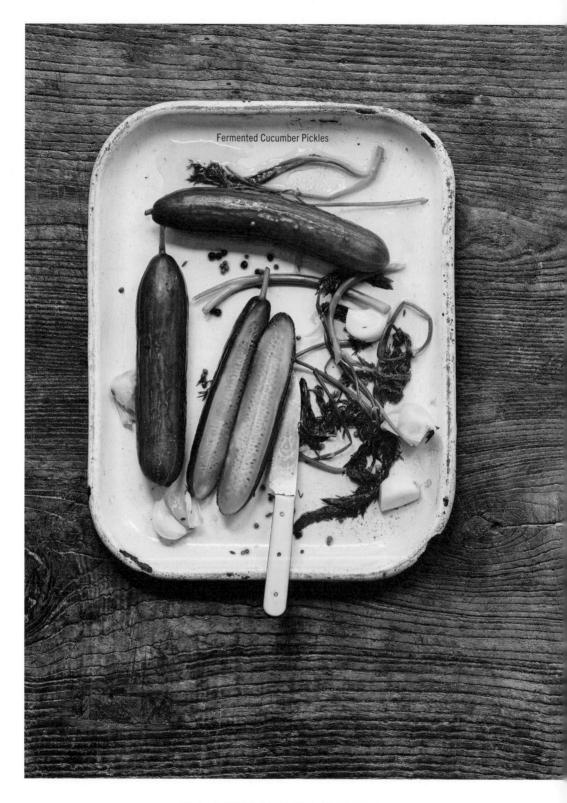

Fermented Cucumber Pickles

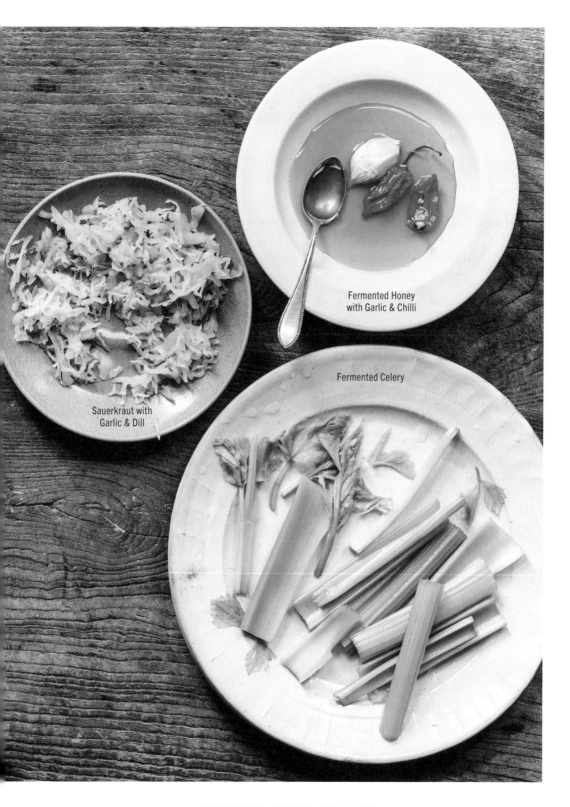

Fermented Honey
with Garlic & Chilli

Fermented Celery

Sauerkraut with
Garlic & Dill

FERMENTED CELERY

Celery is often overlooked as a vegetable in its own right, as it's usually associated with aromatics such as carrots, onions, leeks and garlic, as a flavour base for soups or stocks, and rarely served as a main event.
By fermenting celery, you create a mellow version of it, raw but 'cooked' by the acid it creates in which it bathes; the brine can be used in a salad dressing, béchamel sauce or soup, or as a stock. Arranged on a plate and simply dressed with some of its own brine, a drizzle of good olive oil and a twist of black pepper, you'll have a very special dish. Also try it as a crudité for dips or as a sofrito, as well as in salads, such as the Chicken Salad with Pears, Blue Cheese, Fermented Celery on page 105.

350–400g (12–14oz) celery with leaves

500g (1lb 2oz) water

20g (¾oz) fine natural sea salt

You will need a 1-litre (1¾-pint) clean ice-cream tub or other lidded food storage container.

Wash and drain the celery, then trim the stalks so that they will come just below the rim of your container when standing upright. Pack the container vertically with the celery – you can fill any gaps with some of the trimmings.

Add the measured water to a mixing bowl with the salt and whisk briskly until the salt has dissolved.

Pour the brine over the celery to cover, then ensure it's as fully submerged as possible by following the smaller lidded container method on page 21.

Leave to ferment in your kitchen for about 7–10 days.

Every few days, 'burp' your fermenting celery as directed on page 21.

After 7–10 days, your celery should taste slightly tangy but savoury, with the harshness of the salt somewhat diminished. The fermentation period will vary, depending on the ambient temperature in your kitchen – the warmer it is, the faster the fermentation. When it's to your taste, store the celery in the fridge, where it will keep happily for 2–3 months.

FERMENTED HONEY WITH GARLIC & CHILLI

This is such a good larder resource, standing ready to deliver a natural sweet, garlic-chilli hit whenever you need it. Fermenting honey involves adding water to enable the microbes and yeasts to activate, as neat honey is dense, acidic and therefore antibacterial, which is what gives it such a long shelf life. Unlike many ferments in this book which call for anaerobic fermentation, this recipe relies on naturally occurring microbes both in the air and on the skin of the chilli and garlic to activate the honey. Try it in stir-fries and on pizzas, as well as in dressings, marinades and mayo, and drizzled over strong cheeses. Try the recipe for Chicken Wings with Fermented Honey Sauce on page 150.

340g (11¾oz) jar natural runny honey

2 tablespoons warm water

6 or 7 garlic cloves (about 20g/¾oz in total), unpeeled and bruised or lightly crushed

1 hot red chilli, such as Scotch bonnet, or 2 jalapeño chillies, if less heat is preferred, halved

Pour the honey in a mixing bowl. To get all the remaining honey out of the jar, add the warm water to the almost empty jar, replace the lid tightly and shake well before pouring the watery honey into the bowl. Stir well.

Drop the garlic cloves and chilli or chillies into the bottom of a thoroughly cleaned Vadasz pot or other 400ml (14fl oz) food storage container with a tight-fitting lid, then pour over the honey. You will have some headspace at the top of the pot, which is fine.

Put the lid on the pot or container to cover loosely, leaving a gap so that air can get in. Leave to ferment in a warmish spot in the kitchen. After a month or so, you should get a good result, but do taste and use over the weeks, as the flavour will develop and change – and that's often the best thing about fermented foods!

This is one of those ferments that you can just leave at an ambient temperature without any need to refrigerate.

FERMENTED CRUSHED TOMATOES

As I mentioned in the introduction, we often associate fermentation with foods that have 'gone off' or are 'bad'. Fermented tomatoes exemplify this really well. As a chef, I recall many occasions when tomatoes went off, especially when mixed with onions and garlic. Most memorable were batches of fresh salsa or pico de gallo not chilled sufficiently during hot summer services, exhibiting the now very familiar tell-tale signs: bubbles and solids rising above the juices, alcoholic and yeasty smell, and a sour, tangy and slightly vinegary taste. Ironic, then, that years later I'm trying to harness those same characteristics, as they add value and enhance flavours naturally. But to do that effectively there must be some controls in place so that they don't go too far and spoil.

You can use any type or quantity of tomatoes, but stick to adding 2% of the total weight in salt — especially handy if you have a glut of home-grown fruit. Celery is an inspired additional aromatic and a nod to my very talented friend Olia Hercules's recipe for whole tomatoes spiked with garlic, chilli and celery, which I helped to prepare for her wonderful pop-ups.

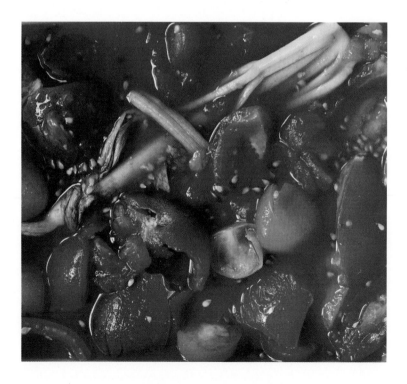

Try these delicious tomatoes as a base for salsas or for a delicious twist on a *pan con tomate* (see page 66), or to create a superior pasta dish, tossed in a pan with good olive oil, some basil leaves, your favourite cooked pasta and plenty of grated Parmesan or pecorino romano. You may need to drain the tomatoes, but make sure you reserve the tomato brine to create a wonderfully flavoured base for dressings, sauces, soups and bloody good Bloody Marys!

1.5kg (3lb 5oz) ripe tomatoes

30g (1oz) fine natural sea salt, or 2% of the total weight of the tomatoes

4 garlic cloves, crushed

1 celery stick with leaves, halved

You will need 2 large lidded plastic food storage containers of the same size, each about 4 litres (7 pints) capacity – thoroughly cleaned ice-cream tubs are perfect.

Wash and drain the tomatoes, then roughly chop and place in a large mixing bowl. Add the salt and garlic and mix well with your hands, squashing and crushing the tomatoes a little to release some of their juices. Now try a little – they should taste saltier than you would like to eat them.

Pack the tomatoes into one of your containers and add the celery halves. Use the second container to submerge your tomatoes fully in their brine, following the weighted second container method on page 20.

Leave to ferment in a corner of your kitchen that has the most even temperature – the ideal range is 15–20°C (59–68°F). Every day, remove the weighted second container to reveal the surface of the fermenting tomatoes – look and listen for bubbling, then taste to experience the transformation from raw to fermented. You will also release any CO_2 build-up from your tomatoes in the process. In a relatively warm kitchen (above 15°C/59°C), they will probably be ready in 3–5 days, possibly only 2 days. As the days pass, you will notice a slight increase in acidity and the harshness of the salt will become more of a savoury note. At this point, before the tomatoes become too fizzy and lively, store in the fridge as they are, or divide between smaller lidded food storage containers. They will keep for 2–3 weeks and will continue to ferment and develop flavour, but much more slowly. If using the small lidded container method, you may need to 'burp' them every 2 days, as directed on page 21.

PINEAPPLE, STRAWBERRY & CUCUMBER SALSA

This is a magical mix of luscious fruit, aromatic herbs and fiery spice. The key to success here is to ferment for just a day or so before transferring to the relative safety of the fridge, as fruit, with its naturally high sugar content, runs the risk of rapidly sending your lacto-fermentation on a one-way ticket to an alcoholic cocktail. Making small batches is therefore a wise move to mitigate the risk of spoilage and wastage. I use this salsa to liven up tacos and tostadas, or serve it ice cold as a spicy fruit or seafood cocktail.

300g (10½oz) fresh pineapple chunks, quartered if large

200g (7oz) strawberries, hulled and quartered

½ cucumber, quartered lengthways and diced

10g (¼oz) fine natural sea salt

juice 1 lime

1 tablespoon gochugaru (Korean red pepper flakes) or pul biber (Aleppo chilli flakes)

1 thumb-sized piece of fresh root ginger, scrubbed and finely chopped

1 garlic clove, crushed

1 red chilli, finely chopped

1 handful of mint, chopped

1 handful of coriander, chopped

Put the fruit and cucumber in a large mixing bowl with the salt and mix gently with your hands.

Add all the remaining ingredients and mix again well with your hands.

Cover the bowl loosely with a clean tea towel and leave the fruit and cucumber mix to macerate for 20 minutes or so.

Pack into thoroughly cleaned Vadasz pots or other 400ml (14fl oz) lidded food storage containers.

Leave to ferment at room temperature for a day or so, checking and tasting regularly for just a hint of fizz before storing in the fridge until needed, where it will keep for a week or so.

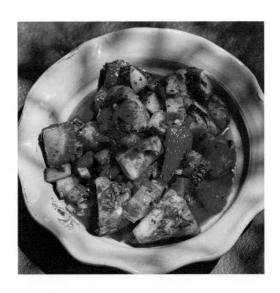

Cold-brined pickles

Unlike the ferments in the previous pages, the recipes in this section are brined in vinegar rather than being allowed to create their own acid. These pickles are generally quicker to make than ferments, and offer bright, zingy flavours and a crunchy texture.

If the salt quantities seem high, bear in mind that a pickle must pack a punch both in its savouriness and acidity. Furthermore, especially if fermenting, the amount of salt must be great enough for it to do its job of drawing out and creating a brine from the natural juices of the vegetables, which acts as an antibacterial agent. I've eaten burgers and sandwiches where the pickle or condiment, lacking enough salt, does nothing to uplift or add value to the dish. A pickle should be transformative and substantial; a purposeful, balancing and supportive addition to the food it's served with.

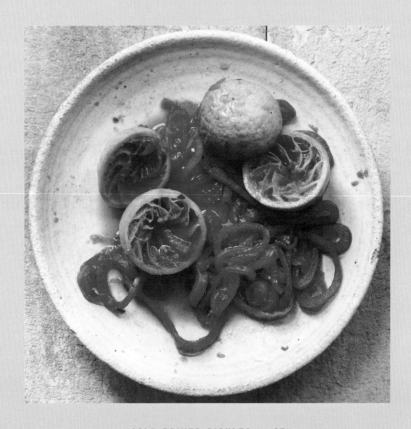

PICKLED RED ONIONS

A favourite across many meals at home, this recipe is a good example of how pickling can be done quickly and easily even without vinegar or salt brine. Here, the necessary acid is provided by the juices of the citrus fruit (limes and pink grapefruit) which is how delicious Mexican *cebolla curtida* (pickled onions) are prepared. This method also draws out and enhances the natural colours of the red onion — like you've just tossed neon strips into your pickles! Use these pickled onions, thinly sliced, in tacos, burritos and sandwiches, or try the Tempura Fried Pickles on page 138, in which case I recommend slicing the onions quite thickly, about 6–7 slices per onion.

3 large red onions

20g (¾oz) fine natural sea salt, or more if needed

4 limes

1 pink grapefruit

1 teaspoon dried oregano (Mexican if possible)

olive oil, to serve (optional)

Trim and peel the onions, then slice thinly into rings for maximum versatility (see introduction above).

Put the red onion slices in a large mixing bowl, cover with the salt and mix together well with your hands.

Set aside to macerate for a few minutes while you halve and squeeze the juice from the limes and grapefruit, reserving the squeezed lime halves.

Add the citrus juices and oregano to the red onion slices and mix well with your hands. Taste and add more salt if needed.

Leave to stand for 10–15 minutes before serving the onions as they are, or with a good swirl or two of olive oil.

To store for later use, pack the pickled onions into a jar or other lidded food storage container, then top with the reserved squeezed lime halves before putting on the lid to help submerge them in the brine. They will keep well in the fridge for a week or so.

PICKLED OKRA

I first made pickled okra for a purely practical reason. One particularly dry summer we were struggling to source enough cucumbers to pickle for my Saturday market stall, so I needed an alternative vegetable. Then I spotted some okra in the market and thought I'd try them. The sliminess of okra can be off-putting, though I personally don't mind it, but I knew that the method in Indian cuisine of salting chopped okra while frying it with onions, garlic and spices drew out moisture and gave a less slimy result. So for those of you who aren't partial to okra's very particular texture, you'll be pleased to hear that pickling delivers a similar result. Not only that, it adds a crunchy bite too. These spicy lady's fingers are perfect for dips — try using them as 'frickles' following the recipe on page 138.

280g (10oz) okra

1 teaspoon coriander seeds

½ teaspoon cumin seeds

½ teaspoon black peppercorns

½ teaspoon nigella seeds

¼ teaspoon ground turmeric

2 garlic cloves, peeled but kept whole

½ long red chilli, halved lengthways

grated zest and juice of ½ lemon

FOR THE BRINE

200g (7oz) apple cider vinegar

80g (2¾oz) water

2 tablespoons sugar

2 teaspoons fine natural sea salt

First make the brine. Put all the ingredients for it in a mixing bowl and whisk briskly to help dissolve the sugar and salt. Don't worry if they don't dissolve completely, as they will continue to dissolve over time in the storage pots.

Wash and drain the okra, then place vertically, stem ends up, in a 1-litre (1¾-pint) deli pot or similar lidded food storage container, or horizontally in 2 thoroughly cleaned Vadasz pots or other 400ml (14fl oz) lidded food storage containers. Add the remaining ingredients, dividing them equally between the pots if using more than one pot.

Pour the brine over the okra to cover. As they brine, they may float up above the surface or there will be some headspace, so ensure that they are as fully submerged as possible by following the smaller lidded container method on page 21.

You can put your okra straight into the fridge to brine slowly, but I usually leave at ambient temperature for a few hours to kick-start the process. Once in the fridge, allow the okra to absorb the spicy brine for at least a week — after 10–14 days you can enjoy your fully flavoured pickled okra. Like all pickles, their flavour and texture will continue to develop over time. They will keep in the fridge for 1–2 months, but I bet you'll eat them before then!

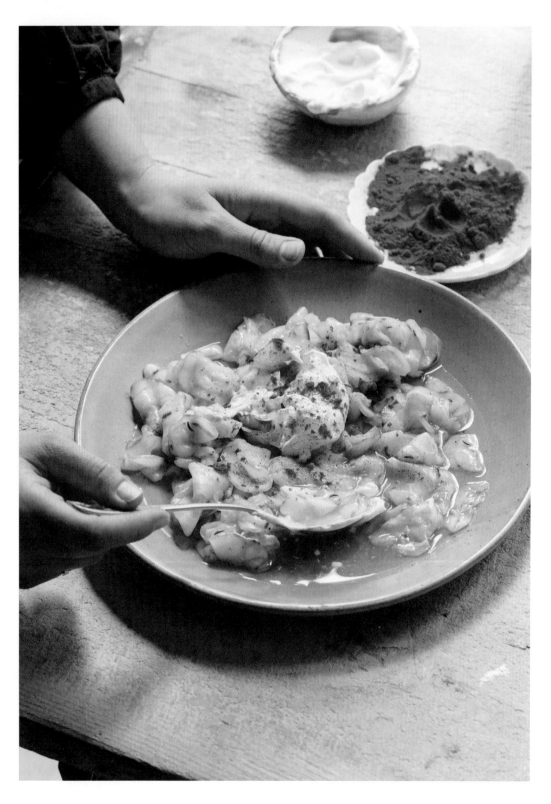

QUICK CUCUMBER PICKLE

Uborka saláta in Hungarian, this is the first pickle I ever made in my grandmother's kitchen (see page 8). It's so simple, yet has such a good flavour — both fresh and pickly — and has served my family and me well for generations. It's my Desert Island pickle for sure, although the Fermented Cucumber Pickles/*kovászos uborka* on page 28 would do me too!. This goes well with the Sabich Pitta, Reuben Sandwich or the Double Pickle Cheeseburger (see pages 75, 79 and 80). Or try enjoying it, well drained, in cucumber sandwiches using very good bread and butter, slicing them up daintily like you're having tea at the Ritz!

3 cucumbers

25g (1oz) fine natural sea salt

FOR THE BRINE

170g (6oz) apple cider vinegar

100g (3½oz) water

2 heaped tablespoons sugar

1 large garlic clove, crushed

1 big pinch of pepper

1 big pinch of caraway seeds

TO SERVE

soured cream

paprika

Wash and drain the cucumbers, then peel them. Using a mandoline or the slicer on your grater, slice the cucumbers thinly.

Put the cucumber slices in a large mixing bowl, cover with the salt and mix well with your hands. You will notice that they begin to lose their juices quickly and diminish in size.

Sit a plate on top of the cucumber slices and leave for 20 minutes or so to draw out the juices even more.

While the cucumber slices are resting in their salty bath, make your brine. Put all the ingredients for it in a separate large mixing bowl and whisk briskly to help dissolve the sugar and salt. Don't worry if they don't dissolve completely, as they will do so during the brining process.

Squeeze the cucumber slices robustly over a colander to remove the excess liquid, then transfer to a salad spinner to expel more of the salty juices. When well and truly squeezed and drained, the cucumber will resemble coin-sized, wilted, pale green jewels. Have a taste, and if you think the cucumbers are too salty, please go ahead and rinse before adding to the vinegar.

Add the cucumber slices to your brine and mix well.

Although the pickle is good to eat straight away, it's best to let the cucumber absorb the brine for at least 20 minutes or so before serving in a bowl topped with soured cream and a dusting of bright red paprika. To store for later use, pack the pickle into 2 thoroughly cleaned Vadasz pots or other 400ml (14fl oz) lidded storage containers and put in the fridge, where it will keep for several weeks.

DO CHUA VIETNAMESE PICKLES

I ate these pickles regularly when I shared a production unit in Hackney with a Vietnamese restaurant. We swapped pickles and cooking ideas, and I soon fell in love with Vietnamese cuisine, especially pho. Crunchy, hot, sweet, sour, spicy and savoury, these pickles are so simple yet so versatile. Be sure to use fresh, firm daikon and carrots — you reap what you sow with pickles! These pickles can be used in the Tofu Banh Mi on page 84 or alongside the Kimchi Special Fried Rice on page 134, or added to soups or scattered through salads. They can even take centre stage in a salad, combined with sliced peppers, spring onions, mint, coriander and more fresh chilli, topped with crushed salted peanuts.

200g (7oz) carrots

700g (1lb 9oz) daikon

1–2 long red chillies, very finely sliced (optional)

FOR THE BRINE

160g (5¾oz) apple cider vinegar

80g (2¾oz) water

80g (2¾oz) sugar

20g (¾oz) fine natural sea salt

First make the brine. Put all the ingredients in a mixing bowl and whisk briskly to help dissolve the sugar and salt. Don't worry if they don't dissolve completely, as they will do so during the brining process.

Wash the carrots and daikon, then trim and peel.

Using a mandoline or the slicer on your grater, slice the vegetables into discs, then cut into fine julienne (long, thin sticks). Alternatively, you could use a julienne peeler or a food processor fitted with a julienne attachment, cutting up the daikon first, as they can be rather large. Place your prepared vegetables in a large mixing bowl.

Give the brine a good final stir, adding the chilli, if using, then pour over the vegetables and mix together by hand to fully combine. Cover loosely with a clean tea towel and leave to brine for a minimum of 1 hour before using.

Pack the pickles into thoroughly cleaned Vadasz pots or other lidded food storage containers and store in the fridge for up to 2 months.

GREEN APPLE CHILLI CHUTNEY

This is a tangy, sweet, sour and spicy quick pickle that you'll want to keep making again and again. It's called a chutney, as it's inspired by the fresh types of Indian chutneys that I've enjoyed so much over the years in east London, served especially, but not exclusively, alongside South Indian dishes, such as dosa and uttapam. Serve it with the chicken curry on page 130; enjoy it on your barbecue menu with handmade lamb koftas or burgers; give it the starring role in a grilled halloumi wrap with garlic and mint yogurt; pack it into a deep-filled mature Cheddar sandwich; slather it on top of a grilled cheese toastie; or use as a base for a grilled vegetable salad.

2 Granny Smith apples, cored, sliced and finely diced

1 forkful of Vadasz Red Onion Pickles or homemade Pickled Red Onions (see page 38)

1 long red chilli, finely diced

1 garlic clove, crushed

1 handful of chopped coriander

1 smaller handful of mint leaves

1 pinch of cumin seeds

1 pinch of nigella seeds

1 tablespoon olive oil

1 teaspoon dark honey

1 teaspoon chilli oil with bits

juice of ½ lime

½ tablespoon apple cider vinegar

1 good pinch each of salt and pepper

Put all the ingredients in a mixing bowl and mix well.

Leave the chutney to stand for a few minutes to allow the flavours to develop before serving.

This is best served freshly made, but any remaining chutney can be stored in the fridge for up to 5 days.

PICKLED FENNEL WITH LEMON

My fennel bulb pickles were always a popular item on the market stalls and also attracted a good number of wholesale customers for sandwiches and for serving with fish. With its pungent liquorice flavour, fennel is one of my favourite vegetables, and it works really well when pickled with lemon. Here, I've given the fennel an extra hit of liquorice with the addition of star anise. Note that fennel will discolour quickly when sliced as it oxidizes, so be sure to add the lemon juice while preparing it. I love to use this delicious pickle in salads, to serve with barbecued pork or sausages, or as the base for a fennel tartar sauce. It also features in the recipe for a tuna and avocado sandwich on page 81 and in Tuna, Mackerel & Onion Bucatini on page 118.

4 fennel bulbs (about 800–900g/
1lb 12oz–2lb in total), fronds attached
if possible

2 lemons, halved

FOR THE BRINE

250g (9oz) apple cider vinegar

125g (4½oz) water

50g (1¾oz) sugar

25g (1oz) fine natural sea salt

2 whole star anise

½ tablespoon coriander seeds

2 teaspoons black peppercorns

First make the brine. Put all the ingredients in a large mixing bowl and whisk briskly until the sugar and salt have dissolved.

Wash and drain the fennel bulbs. Using a sharp knife, the slicer on your grater, or a food processor fitted with a thin slicer attachment, slice the fennel very finely, squeezing a lemon half over each bulb as you slice it. Reserve the squeezed lemon halves.

Add the fennel to the brine and mix well.

Pack the pickle into a few thoroughly cleaned Vadasz pots or other lidded food storage containers. Flatten-out the reserved squeezed lemon halves and place them on top of the fennel to impart more lemon flavour and help submerge them in the brine before putting on the lids. This will keep for several weeks in the fridge, but can be used after just 1–2 hours as a deliciously fresh pickle.

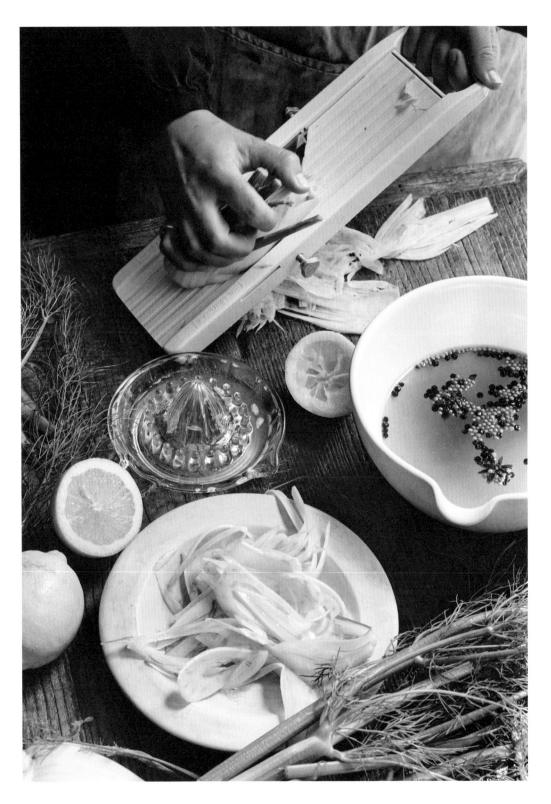

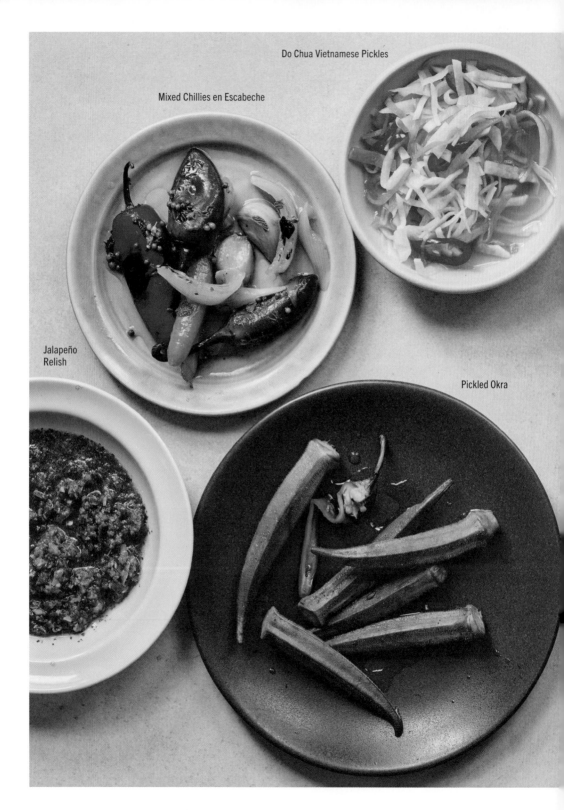

Do Chua Vietnamese Pickles

Mixed Chillies en Escabeche

Jalapeño
Relish

Pickled Okra

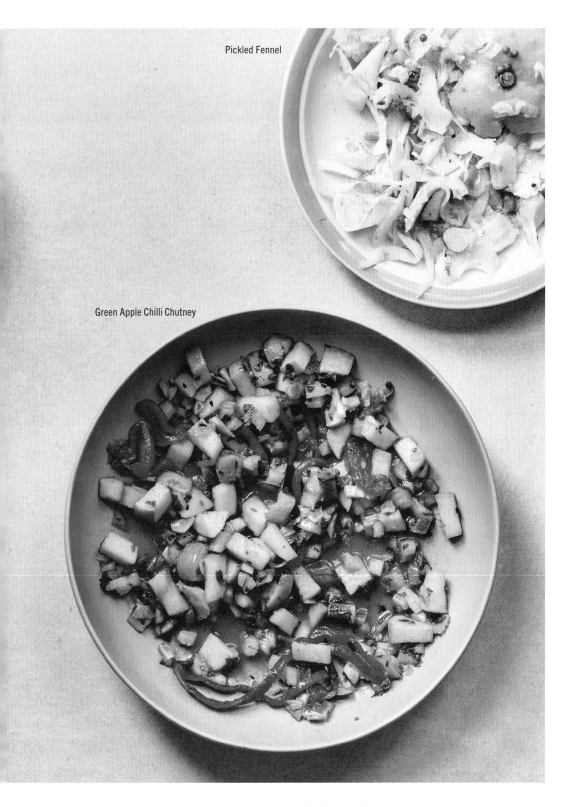

Pickled Fennel

Green Apple Chilli Chutney

MIXED CHILLIES EN ESCABECHE

I first fell in love with these pickles years ago as a chef when serving them as a side in a Mexican restaurant. Later, they made a regular appearance on my pickle stall at the street markets across London. I love how the heat is mellowed and tempered by the acid of the vinegar, along with the onions and garlic. There is a lovely fragrant aroma from the oregano, and the carrots give both texture and colour. You can use up any surplus chillies to make this, but I prefer to stick to larger, milder ones such as jalapeño, serenade or cayenne. These chillies can be used in the Tofu Banh Mi recipe on page 84, and also make a great addition to salads, fried eggs, cheese on toast or quesadillas and refried beans.

½ tablespoon olive oil

8–12 (about 200g/7oz in total) whole jalapeño chillies or other large mixed mild chillies

1 small onion, halved and sliced into semicircles

1 small carrot, peeled and sliced at an angle

3 garlic cloves, unpeeled

1 big pinch of dried oregano (Mexican if possible)

2 teaspoons fine natural sea salt

½ teaspoon cumin seeds

½ teaspoon coriander seeds

FOR THE BRINE

apple cider vinegar (see method)

water (see method)

Heat the olive oil in a skillet or heavy-based frying pan over a high heat. When hot, sear the whole chillies with the onion, carrot and garlic for a few minutes, turning frequently until evenly blistered and charred. Transfer them to a bowl and leave to cool slightly.

Spoon into a thoroughly clean used Vadasz pot or other 400–500ml (14–18fl oz) lidded food storage container, along with the oregano, salt and spices.

To make the brine, fill your pot two-thirds full with the vinegar and one-third full with water to cover. Put the lid on tightly and turn over a few times to mix the brine and all the ingredients together.

Store your pickle pot in a cool corner of the kitchen, if you want to use within a week or so, or store in the fridge where it will keep for 3–4 months. You can start to eat the chillies after just a few hours, but they will be at their best after 1–2 weeks.

JALAPEÑO RELISH

My original recipe was for a cooked relish thickened with cornflour. It was very good but predated my progression to cold-brining pickles, so I adapted the recipe and it's all the better for that. This is a hot, spicy, super-quick chilli relish, sweeter and spicier than the Mixed Chillies en Escabeche (opposite), and one that works so well with the Mexican dishes in Part Two such as Green Eggs & Ham on Toast on page 59 and Tortilla Chips with Fresh Salsa & Eggs on page 64, as well as the South and East Asian recipes, though I challenge you not to add it to almost everything you eat. Make sure you chop all the veggies small enough to allow them to blend easily and evenly.

FOR THE RELISH

8–12 mixed red and green chillies, chopped

2 green peppers, cored, deseeded and chopped

2 small onions, chopped

4 garlic cloves, peeled but kept whole

1 bunch of coriander, roughly chopped

FOR THE BRINE & SEASONING

100g (3½oz) apple cider vinegar

2 tablespoons olive oil

½ teaspoon cumin seeds

½ teaspoon coriander seeds

½ teaspoon ground turmeric

10g (¼oz) fine natural sea salt

1 tablespoon sugar

Put all the ingredients for the relish in the large bowl of a food processor and pulse until you have a fine texture — you might need to do this in batches, depending on the size of your machine.

Empty the relish into a large mixing bowl, add all the ingredients for the brine and seasoning and mix well to combine. Taste for salt, adding more if needed.

Transfer the relish to a lidded food storage container. You can use straight away and store the remainder in the fridge, where it will keep for a month.

Part Two

USING PICKLES & FERMENTS

BREAKFAST
& BRUNCH

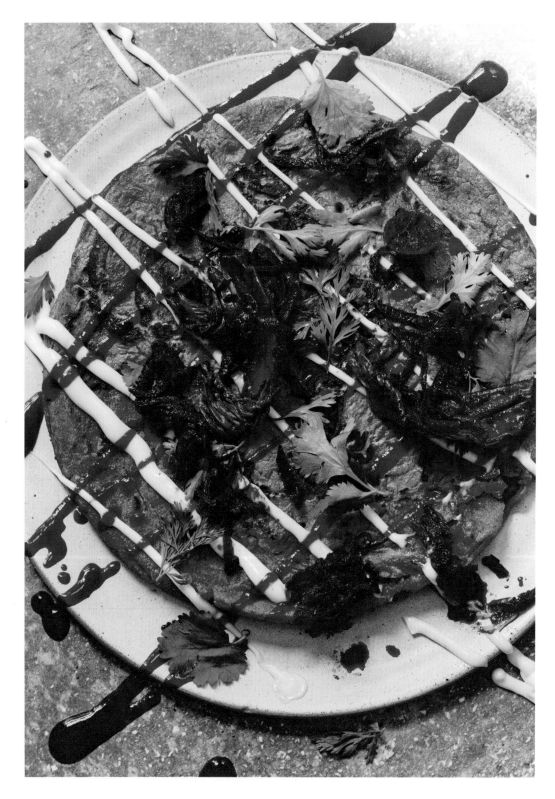

SUPER-BEET KIMCHI PANCAKE WITH PURPLE SRIRACHA

Kimchi pancakes are a must when you're eating out at a Korean restaurant. In my version here, I use our Vadasz Super-Beet Kimchi to add some purple haze to my days! You can go wild with the garnish and add even more vibrant colour: pile it high with a chopped fresh salad or a homemade slaw, or top with a fried egg and some feta or mozzarella cheese.

75g (2¾oz) gram (chickpea) flour

¼ teaspoon baking powder

80ml (2¾fl oz) water

150g (5½oz) Vadasz Super-Beet Kimchi or homemade Beetroot Kimchi (see page 25), plus extra to garnish

2 tablespoons olive oil

TO GARNISH

1 tablespoon sriracha sauce mixed with 1½ tablespoons of the beetroot kimchi brine

a squirt of mayonnaise

1 big pinch of chopped coriander

Mix the flour and baking powder together in a bowl, then gradually stir in the water until you have a smooth batter. Add the beetroot kimchi and mix well to incorporate.

Heat the olive oil in a large frying pan over a medium hea. When hot, ladle or pour the batter in, rotating and tilting the pan to ensure the batter is evenly spread — you might need to give it a nudge with a spatula to encourage it to spread out.

Cook for 4 minutes until the edges of the pancake just begin to crisp and brown, then carefully flip, using a spatula if necessary, and cook for another minute or so before sliding on to a serving plate.

Now build your garnish. Sprinkle more of the beetroot kimchi liberally over the top of the pancake and follow with zigzags of the purple sriracha and mayo. Lastly, scatter over the chopped coriander. Cut into 6, like a pizza, to serve.

CHEESE & PICKLE BREAKFAST QUESADILLA

Quesadillas make the perfect quick breakfast, brunch or snack. While the marriage of cheese and tortilla (flour or corn) is, of course, the foundation of a quesadilla, it's the additional punch from pickles and ferments that elevates this savoury staple. Here I've kept it simple but delicious by using Jalapeño relish or pickled red onions, but you can easily swap those out for Vadasz Kimchi or your homemade kimchi (see page 24). Try the various options and decide which is your go-to favourite. Oh, and you can also add tomatoes, ham or cooked chorizo, bacon or mushrooms — all work really well. This takes just a flash to cook, so get your ingredients ready to roll before you start.

olive oil

2 eggs

½ small onion, finely diced

1 big handful of grated Cheddar cheese, or a mix of chopped mozzarella and crumbled feta cheese

1 large flour or corn tortilla/wrap

1 forkful of Vadasz Jalapeño Relish or homemade Jalapeño Relish (see page 49), or Vadasz Red Onion Pickles or homemade Pickled Red Onions (see page 38)

½ avocado, peeled and sliced

salt and pepper

TO SERVE

a splash of your favourite hot sauce (optional)

a smear of soured cream

1 lime wedge

Heat a large, heavy-based frying pan over a medium heat and add a drizzle of olive oil, ensuring the base is completely covered.

Beat the eggs with the onion in a bowl and season with salt and pepper. Pour into the hot pan, rotating and tilting to cover the base with the egg mixture but leaving a border of a few centimetres (an inch or so) around the edge.

Immediately sprinkle the cheese over the egg, ensuring some is distributed on to the pan beyond the edge of the omelette to create a cheesy crust. Take the pan off the heat — the omelette won't be fully cooked at this stage, but the residual heat will finish the job.

Toast the tortilla directly over the open flame of your gas hob, if you have one, or in a hot, dry frying pan for a few seconds on one side only, being careful not to burn it — you want it to blister and brown a little but not too much.

Lay the tortilla, toasted side facing up, in the palm of one hand, then slap it down on top of the omelette and, applying some pressure, swivel it to loosen the omelette from the pan (like you're a seasoned DJ on the turntables, scratching away like it's back in the day!). Carefully invert the contents of the pan back into your palm, then deftly slide it back into the pan, tortilla side down, to toast the other side — you might need to use a spatula and a plate to do this.

Return the pan to the heat, add your relish or pickles and avocado to one half and fold the other half over to cover. Continue to cook for 1 minute before sliding the quesadilla out on to a chopping board.

Cut into triangles and serve with hot sauce, if you like, a touch of soured cream and the lime wedge.

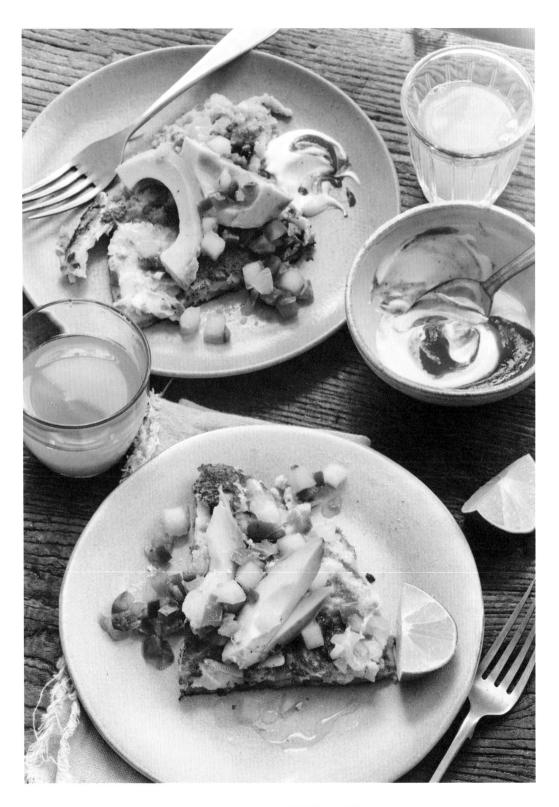

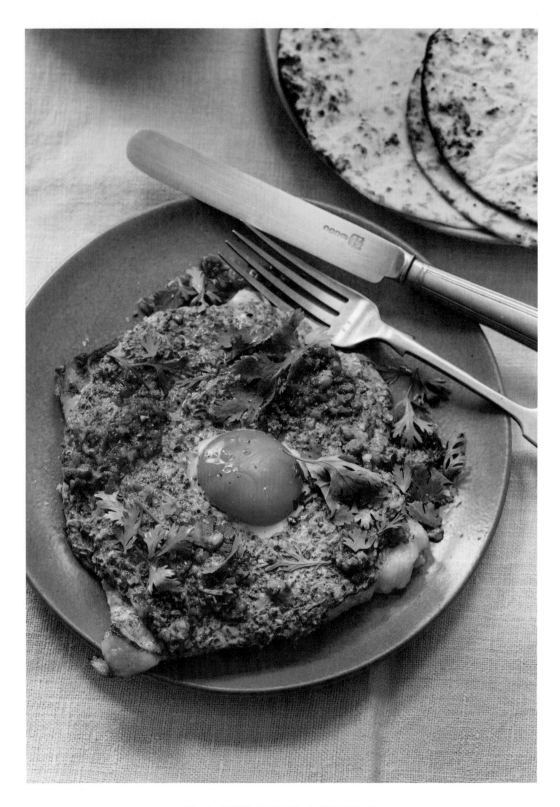

GREEN EGGS & HAM

Dr Seuss's Sam-I-Am famously did not like green eggs and ham, but if he had added some jalapeño relish, I'm sure he'd have eaten them here or there, he'd have eaten them anywhere!

60g (2½oz) baby spinach

20g (¾oz) kale, chopped

5 spring onions, sliced

1 garlic clove, chopped

1 tablespoon Vadasz Jalapeño Relish brine or homemade Jalapeño Relish brine (see page 49), or any other pickle brine you have at hand

2 eggs, whites and yolks separated into 2 small bowls (take care to keep the yolks intact)

a big blob of butter

2 thick slices of quality ham — enough to roughly cover the base of your frying pan

1 or 2 corn or flour tortillas

salt and pepper

TO GARNISH

1 tablespoon Vadasz Jalapeño Relish or homemade Jalapeño Relish (see page 49)

1 big pinch of chopped coriander

a swirl or two of good olive oil

Put the spinach, kale, spring onions, garlic, brine, egg whites and some salt and pepper in a food processor or a blender and pulse until you have a smooth green batter — it will thicken slightly from the egg whites. Scrape into a bowl.

Heat the butter n a frying pan with a lid over a low to medium heat, rotating and tilting the pan to ensure the base and sides are coated with melted butter. Add the ham and fry gently on one side only for 2 minutes, shaking the pan every few seconds.

Make sure the slices of ham are covering the base of the pan, then spoon half the green batter over them and use the back of the spoon to spread it evenly. Cover the pan and cook very gently for 2–3 minutes.

Now carefully slide the yolks on top of the batter in the centre of each slice of ham, then replace the lid and cook for 1½ minutes. Take the pan off the heat and leave to rest for 2 minutes, keeping the lid on. The yolks might not look completely done yet but they'll continue to cook as they sit.

Remove the lid — the yolks should still be runny and the batter softly set. Run a flexible spatula around the edge of the green batter, then lift and slide it and the ham on to a warm serving plate, taking care not to break the yolks. Garnish with the jalapeño relish and coriander, finishing with a swirl or two of good olive oil.

Toast the tortillas directly over the naked flame of your gas hob, if you have one, or in a hot, dry frying pan for a few seconds on each side, until warmed and slightly charred. Serve with the green eggs and ham for dipping and scooping it all up.

KIMCHEESE BEANS ON TOAST

The pairing of savoury, tangy, spicy kimchi and strong, creamy Cheddar cheese has long been a favourite of mine and has now become popular among kimchi lovers everywhere. Here, I've combined that winning formula with possibly the UK's favourite snack: beans on toast. Done right, you'll have a wonderful balance of crunchy parts of the toast that have held up well to the cheesy kimchi beans, and softer parts that have been swamped by the sauce, absorbing all its delicious flavour.

2 thick slices of good-quality white or wholemeal sourdough bread

415g (14¾oz) can baked beans

2 tablespoons Vadasz Kimchi or homemade Kimchi (see page 24), plus 1 tablespoon to garnish

60g (2¼oz) mature Cheddar cheese, grated, plus 1 big pinch to garnish

1 teaspoon butter, plus extra for the toasted bread

1–2 spring onions, finely sliced

Toast the bread in a toaster, twice if necessary to get the required doneness needed to hold the beans, then leave in the toaster to help retain its crunch.

While the bread is toasting, heat a wide nonstick frying pan over a medium heat.

Empty the beans into a saucepan over a medium heat and begin to heat, adding the kimchi, half the cheese and the 1 teaspoon butter. Stir briskly and heat for about 6 minutes until the mixture is bubbling and thickening.

While the beans are heating up, add a little of the extra butter to the hot frying pan, spreading it over the base. As soon as it's melted, add the remaining cheese, covering the entire base of the pan, immediately followed by the toasted bread slices. Push them down with your fingers and then from side to side, which will loosen the cheese from the pan and attach it to the toast as you apply pressure. After 1–2 minutes, or when the cheese has melted and gained some colour, use a firm spatula to shovel the cheesy toasts on to 2 plates, cheesy side up.

The beans will now be bubbling hot, thick and creamy. Spoon them generously over each cheesy toast, then top with the extra grated cheese and kimchi, and sprinkle over the spring onions.

CURRIED SCRAMBLED EGGS ON TOAST

Fried, poached or scrambled? I can never decide! On this occasion, though, I decided I wanted to make scrambled eggs with the Vadasz Pineapple & Turmeric Sauerkraut — something luscious and spicy, yet light, almost soufflé-like in texture. This recipe demonstrates again how versatile sauerkraut is, boldly going where no sauerkraut has been before. Instead of the toast, try serving the eggs with flatbreads, naans or muffins, which would all work nicely too.

100g (3½oz) Vadasz Pineapple & Turmeric Sauerkraut or homemade Curried Kraut (see page 27), plus a little extra to serve

3 eggs

20g (¾oz) butter, plus extra for buttering the toast

2 slices of thick white bread

a drizzle of single cream

2 spring onions, finely sliced

salt and pepper

Drain your sauerkraut in a sieve and squeeze out the brine until thoroughly dry. You can save the brine for using in salad dressings or stock for curries.

Put the sauerkraut in a food processor or a blender and pulse until as smooth as you can get it — you might need to scrape down the sides of the bowl several times to achieve this.

Beat the eggs in a bowl. Add the sauerkraut purée, season with salt and pepper and mix together gently — don't beat.

Heat the butter in a saucepan over a low heat. When hot, add the egg and sauerkraut mixture and cook gently, stirring continuously, for about 3–4 minutes, until starting to firm up and thicken. You want a very soft scramble, with the heat from the butter cooking the eggs rather than the base of the pan, so take the pan off the heat while they are still too soft, as the residual heat will do the rest of the cooking.

Meanwhile, toast your bread and spread with butter.

Swirl the cream and spring onions through the eggs before pouring them on to the toast and topping with a flash more of tangy yellow sauerkraut.

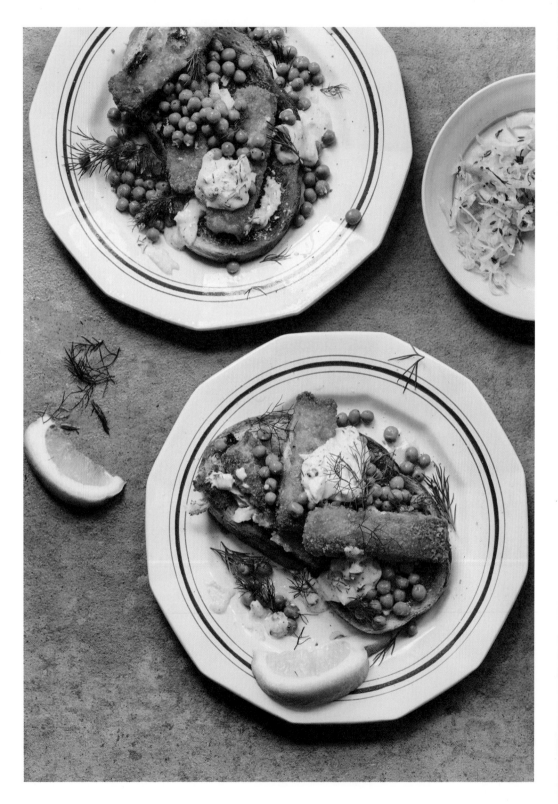

FISH FINGERS & PEAS ON TOAST WITH SAUCE GRIBICHE

Rich yet agreeably acidic, gribiche is a great way to dress anything from poached salmon to cold roast pork, or for dipping tender spears of cooked fresh asparagus when in season. But nothing beats my fish fingers and peas on toast smothered with this simply delicious sauce.

4–6 fresh or frozen fish fingers

a blob of butter, plus extra for buttering the toast

2 handfuls of frozen peas – petit pois are best

2 slices of thick white bread – bloomer or similar, or even sourdough, but not too chewy, holey or challenging on the bite

salt and pepper

2 lemon wedges, to garnish

FOR THE SAUCE GRIBICHE
(makes about 180g/6¼oz)

1 large egg

½ tablespoon Dijon mustard

½ tablespoon white wine vinegar

40g (1½oz) Vadasz Garlic & Dill Sauerkraut or homemade Sauerkraut with Garlic & Dill (see page 26)

75ml (2½fl oz) olive oil

1 tablespoon capers, drained

1 big pinch of chopped dill, plus extra to garnish

First make the gribiche. Bring a small saucepan of water to the boil, add the egg and boil for 8 minutes. Using a slotted spoon, transfer immediately to a bowl of cold water. When cool enough to handle, shell the egg, cut in half and scoop out the yolk, reserving the white.

Put the yolk in the small bowl of a food processor or a blender with the mustard, vinegar, sauerkraut and a pinch each of salt and pepper. Blend together and then, with the machine running, drizzle in the olive oil slowly until emulsified, like a mayo. Transfer to a bowl. Chop the egg white and add to the sauce along with the capers and dill. Season to taste with salt and pepper.

Cover with clingfilm and store in the fridge until you are ready to use it – it should keep well for 5 days or so, but is best enjoyed at room temperature the same day you make it. If you've pre-made the sauce, remove from the fridge at least an hour before serving, if possible, to bring to room temperature.

Cook your fish fingers according to the packet instructions.

Meanwhile, add the butter to a small saucepan with the peas, season with salt and pepper and gently stir and heat up until defrosted and warmed through.

Toast the bread in a toaster, then leave in the toaster for a few minutes before you spread with butter, to help retain its crunch.

Arrange the buttered toast on plates, lay the fish fingers on top and spoon the buttery peas over them. Add generous dollops of the gribiche and garnish each serving with a little extra dill and a lemon wedge.

TORTILLA CHIPS WITH FRESH SALSA & EGGS

Somewhere in the world between a shakshuka and chilaquiles lives this really satisfying brunch dish, where whole eggs are broken on to a stack of fried tortilla chips, which are simmering in a lovely fresh jalapeño relish salsa, creating a soft pie that's formed as the salsa is absorbed by the chips. Done right, it retains some crispy textures too.

1 tablespoon olive oil

170–200g (6–7oz) bag plain tortilla chips

4 eggs

1 handful of grated Cheddar or mozzarella cheese

FOR THE SALSA

4 large ripe tomatoes

1 red pepper, halved, cored and deseeded

1 onion, halved and peeled

2 garlic cloves, unpeeled

2 tablespoons olive oil

1 tablespoon Vadasz Jalapeño Relish or homemade Jalapeño Relish (see page 49)

salt and pepper

TO SERVE

4 tablespoons Vadasz Jalapeño Relish or homemade Jalapeño Relish (see page 49)

2 tablespoons soured cream

4 pinches of chopped coriander

4 lime wedges

First make the salsa. Heat a large frying pan over a medium-high heat, add the tomatoes, red pepper, onion and garlic and cook for about 5–6 minutes, until you have good blackened patches on all the vegetables.

Take the pan off the heat. When cool enough to handle, peel the garlic, add to a food processor or blender with the other charred vegetables, the olive oil, jalapeño relish and some salt and pepper, and blend until you have a smooth salsa.

Add the 1 tablespoon olive oil to the frying pan, followed by the salsa, and bring to a very gentle simmer. Add the tortilla chips, stirring just enough to submerge some but not all of them. Break the eggs on to the chips at quarter intervals around the pan to create portions when you come to serve it, then sprinkle with the cheese.

Cover the pan and cook the eggs very gently — they should cook both from the salsa beneath them and the steam above them under the lid. Check to see if they are done after 3–4 minutes. I like to have soft yolks, but make sure the whites are firm.

Using a large spatula, shovel the portions on to warmed plates and garnish each with a tablespoonful of jalapeño relish, ½ a tablespoonful soured cream, a pinch of chopped coriander and a lime wedge.

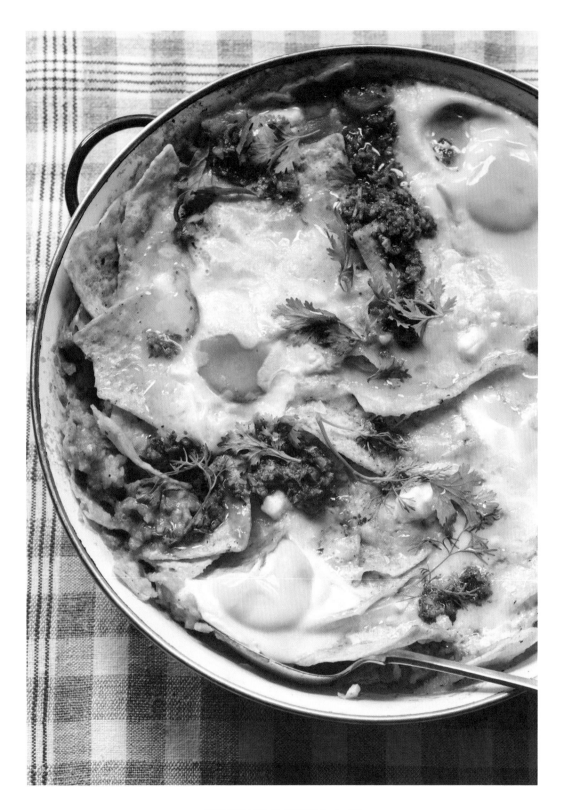

FERMENTED TOMATOES ON TOAST

A classic crowd-pleaser of simple, perfectly seasoned, olive oil-glossed chopped tomatoes and garlic on toast — how do you make something as good as *pan con tomate* even better? Ferment your tomatoes, of course!

good olive oil

1 thick slice of sourdough bread

½ garlic clove, peeled (optional)

2–3 heaped tablespoons Fermented Crushed Tomatoes (see page 34), drained

salt and pepper

Heat a large skillet or heavy-based frying pan over a medium heat.

While the pan is heating up, drizzle plenty of olive oil over both sides of the bread.

Add the bread to the hot pan and toast for about 2 minutes on each side, until golden brown.

Transfer the toast to a chopping board. Rub the garlic clove, if using, all over the toast, especially along the edges, which will impart more garlic flavour. Season with salt.

Spoon the tomatoes on to the toast, then slice in half, place on a plate and add a big swirl of the olive oil and a pinch of pepper.

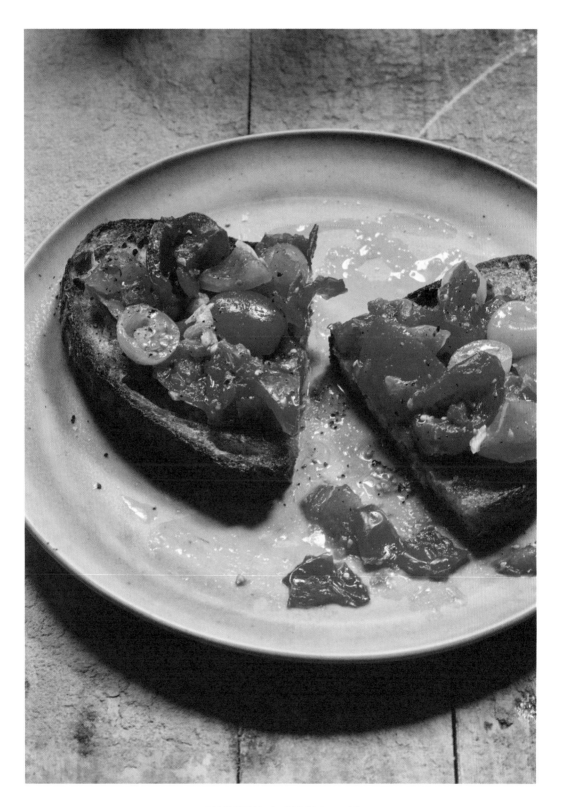

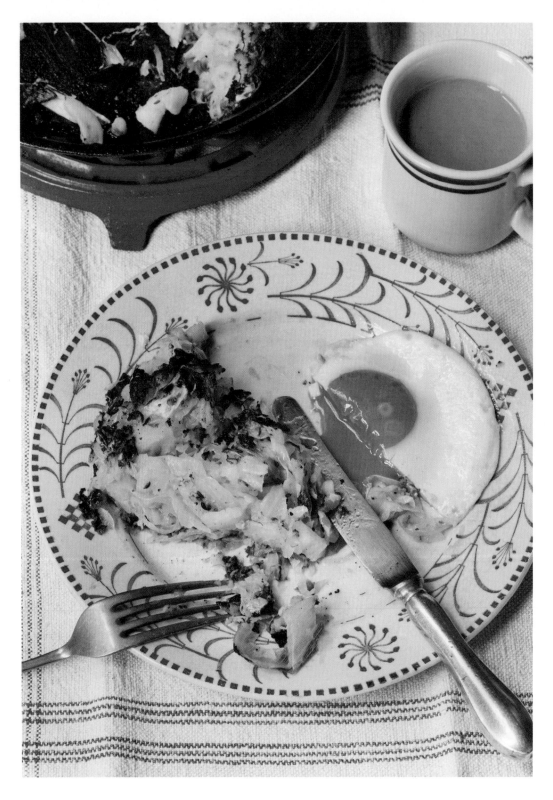

BUBBLE & SQUEAK WITH SAUERKRAUT

Most of us would agree that nothing tastes better in this world than fried or roasted potatoes. But one of my favourite things to eat is bubble and squeak, where leftover cooked potatoes and cabbage are combined into a rough mash and fried slowly and thoroughly until it catches on the surface of the pan and layers of crust are formed. Here, I've pepped up the classic approach with the addition of sauerkraut. While it's delicious simply topped with fried eggs, you can go all out and top with all or any of the other components of the traditional 'full English breakfast': bacon, sausage, beans, tomatoes and so on. If you're cooking bacon, be sure not to waste its precious rendered fat — use it for frying up the bubble and squeak.

500g (1lb 2oz) white potatoes, such as Maris Piper, or baking potatoes

200g (7oz) Vadasz Garlic & Dill Sauerkraut or homemade Sauerkraut with Garlic & Dill (see page 26)

100g (3½oz) leftover cooked vegetables, such as cabbage, peas and leeks

2 spring onions, finely sliced

10g (¼oz) butter

2 tablespoons vegetable oil

4 eggs

salt and pepper

Peel the potatoes, then halve or quarter them if necessary so that they are roughly the same size. Rinse to remove the excess starch, drain and put in a large pan. Cover with cold salted water, bring to the boil and cook for about 15 minutes.

While the potatoes are cooking, put the sauerkraut, cooked vegetables and spring onions in a large mixing bowl and mix well.

When the potatoes are ready — they should be soft enough to break when prodded with a fork but still retain some texture — drain well and let them steam-dry in the colander for a couple of minutes. Then add to the mixing bowl along with the butter and some salt and pepper. Using a fork, mix with the sauerkraut mixture, beating vigorously for just a few seconds to create a mash, but ensuring you retain some bigger pieces too.

Heat the vegetable oil in a heavy-based frying pan over a medium heat. When hot, carefully add the potato mixture, pressing down and spreading it out across the base of the pan until it's completely covered. Leave it to bubble and squeak for 8–10 minutes.

Using 2 firm spatulas, begin to form the potato mixture into 4 roughly rectangular patties, pushing, rotating and shaping. As you do so, you will create more crust. Once you have formed your patties, turn each of them over with the spatulas to cook on the other side for another 8–10 minutes — don't worry if they don't stay together, as you can always re-form them. You want to get a good crust but you don't want them to burn, so keep the temperature on medium-high. Transfer the bubble and squeak patties on to 4 warmed serving plates.

Quickly fry the eggs to your liking in the frying pan and place one on top of each bubble and squeak patty.

SANDWICHES

GRILLED KIMCHEESE

I discovered the joy of melting cheese and kimchi before these toasties became such a popular item on the menus of busy cafés and street-food stalls as they are today — one of life's great pleasures. This has got to be the ultimate and most indulgent grilled kimcheese sandwich, with its combo of kimchi, garlic and herb cream cheese and grated Cheddar to conquer all contenders.

100g (3½oz) Vadasz Kimchi or homemade Kimchi (see page 24), plus extra (or a pickle or two of your choice), to serve

1 tablespoon Boursin or other garlic and herb cream cheese

70g (2½oz) mature Cheddar cheese, grated

a big blob of butter

2 slices of good-quality sourdough bread

Put the kimchi, cream cheese and Cheddar in a mixing bowl and mix well.

Melt the butter in a large, heavy-based frying pan over a very gentle heat. Add the bread and toast lightly for 1–2 minutes on each side — you want the bread to absorb the butter but not toast too much.

When the butter has been absorbed, begin to build the sandwich in the pan, loading on and then spreading the kimcheese mixture on to one bread slice, placing the other slice on top and using a spatula to press it down. For the best gooey/grilled results, lay a piece of folded baking paper or foil over the sandwich and sit a small heavy-based pan on top (I use an antique iron, but you can choose anything heavy.)

Keep the heat low to medium as the sandwich grills so that it builds up a good crisp texture and flavour. After a few minutes, check the underside to ensure it has just the right amount of colour and crispness, then turn the sandwich over. You should hear the reassuring sound of sizzling, oozing, melting cheese and the occasional pop of steam as the kimchi brine hits the hot pan, but it's the unmistakable smell of kimcheese that will get you salivating the most!

Once the bread is deeply golden and toasted on the other side and the cheese has melted, shovel it out of the hot pan, capturing all those lovely charred bits, onto a chopping board and slice in half. Stack on a plate with some more kimchi or one or two of your favourite pickles.

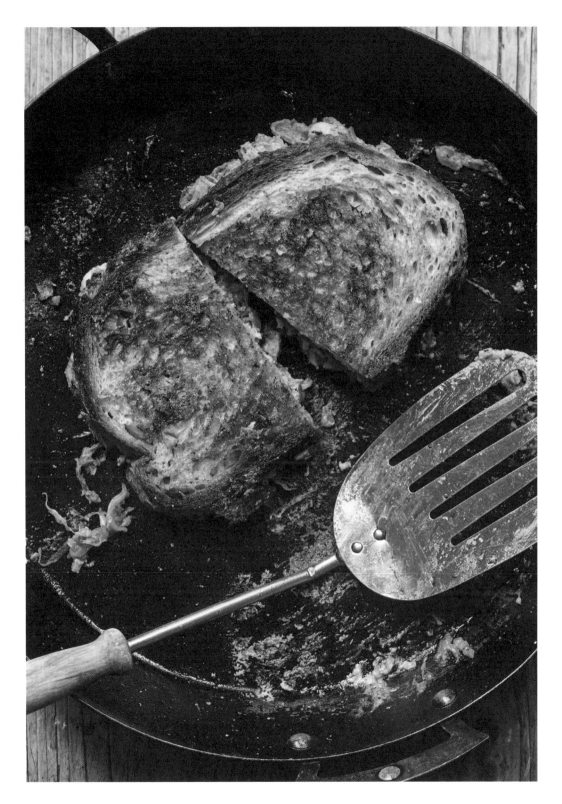

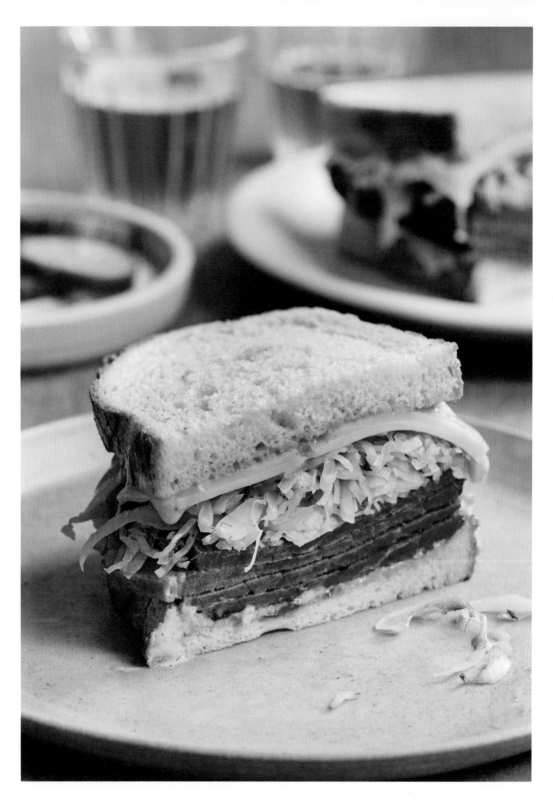

REUBEN SANDWICH

Back in the day, on my way to Brockley Market in southeast London, I would stop off at Druid Street to deliver my Garlic & Dill Sauerkraut to Monty's Deli, where they used it to fill their famous Reubens. Mark and Owen were masters at creating some of the best salt beef around, so I was pretty proud that they used my sauerkraut. I always liked to keep my customers happy, so when they requested I squeezed out all the brine before packing the kraut, I agreed: there's a fine line between a juicy sandwich and a soggy one! This is my version of one of the world's most iconic sandwiches.

vegetable oil, for frying

200g (7oz) corned beef, pastrami or salt beef slices

100g (3½oz) Vadasz Garlic & Dill Sauerkraut or homemade Sauerkraut with Garlic & Dill (see page 26), squeezed out until dry, reserving the brine

2 slices of Emmental cheese

2 thin slices of caraway or rye bread, or a good-quality soft white bread (but not sourdough)

pepper

FOR THE RUSSIAN DRESSING

2 tablespoons mayonnaise

1 tablespoon mustard – a mix of Dijon and American works best

1 tablespoon Vadasz Super-Beet Kimchi brine or homemade Beetroot Kimchi brine (see page 25)

1 teaspoon horseradish sauce

1 tablespoon very finely diced onions

1 tablespoon very finely diced red pepper

1 or 2 slices of Vadasz Garlic & Dill Pickles or homemade Quick Cucumber Pickle (see page 41), plus extra to serve

½ garlic clove, crushed

½ teaspoon paprika

salt and pepper, if needed

First make your Russian dressing. Put all the ingredients in a bowl and mix well. Taste and add salt and pepper, if needed. (Any leftover dressing can be stored in the fridge for up to 5 days.)

Heat a large heavy-based frying pan over a low to medium heat. Once warmed up, cover the base with a few drops of vegetable oil. Carefully add the beef slices to one side of the pan and cook very gently for 2–3 minutes, until heated through, seasoning well with plenty of pepper.

Top the beef with the sauerkraut, followed by the cheese. With a pan lid at the ready, pour a little of the reserved sauerkraut brine into the pan. As this starts to sizzle, immediately cover to harness the steam, which will melt the cheese in just a few seconds. Remove the cover and voilà!

Place one bread slice in the pan next to the beef/kraut/cheese and spread some of the dressing on it. Using a good firm spatula, shovel the beef/kraut/cheese on to the bread. Add the second bread slice to the pan where the beef/kraut/cheese had been and spread with the dressing too. Turn the heat off and top the sandwich with the second bread slice, dressing side down.

Using the spatula, carefully lift the sandwich out of the pan onto a chopping board. Holding the sandwich firmly, position the blade of your most reliably sharp knife across the middle and slice the sandwich in half (I find a serrated bread knife is best: less pressure needed, so less chance of collapse.) Stack your reuben on a plate and serve with a side of cucumber pickles and plenty of kitchen paper!

TANDOORI-STYLE CHICKEN ROLLS WITH PINEAPPLE CURRY KRAUT

This is my homemade version of our family favourite go-to Friday night takeaway, and a very popular one it is too! But if you really, really insist on a takeaway instead, be sure to open it up and 'Vadaszle' it with our Pineapple & Turmeric Sauerkraut or homemade Curried Kraut, then rewrap and devour!

4 large boneless, skinless chicken thighs

FOR THE MARINADE

2 heaped tablespoons Vadasz Pineapple & Turmeric Sauerkraut or homemade Curried Kraut (see page 27), plus extra to serve

2 tablespoons Greek yogurt

1 teaspoon tomato purée

2 teaspoons paprika

2 garlic cloves, crushed

1 handful of chopped coriander, plus ½ handful extra to serve

2 tablespoons olive oil

1 or 2 big pinches of salt and pepper

FOR THE CURRY KETCHUP

2 tablespoons tomato ketchup

1 tablespoon Vadasz Pineapple & Turmeric Sauerkraut or homemade Curried Kraut (see page 27), finely chopped, plus 2 tablespoons of the brine

½ teaspoon sriracha

salt, if needed

TO SERVE

2 large white or wholemeal wraps or fresh naan

a good squirt of mayonnaise

½ handful of chopped mint

juice of ½ lemon

First make your curry ketchup. Put all the ingredients for it in a small bowl and mix well. Taste and add salt if needed.

Place the chicken thighs in a bowl. Put all the marinade ingredients in a food processor or a blender and blend until smooth. Add this to the chicken and mix well to coat. Cover the bowl with clingfilm and leave the chicken to marinate in the fridge for at least 2 hours, but overnight is best.

Preheat the oven to 220°C/200°C fan (425°F), Gas Mark 7. Place the marinated chicken thighs in a baking tray and bake for 20–25 minutes or until well browned and cooked through (if using a probe thermometer, the temperature should be above 74°C/165°F). You might need to adjust the timings depending on how big your thighs are. Turn them over halfway through to get a good even colour on them.

Remove the chicken from the oven, transfer to a bowl or plate and leave to rest for a few minutes.

While the chicken is resting, cut 4 large pieces of greaseproof paper or foil and place on your work surface. Toast each of the wraps or naans directly over the open flame of your gas hob or in a hot, dry frying pan for a few seconds on each side, until warmed and slightly charred. Lay each flat on the paper or foil and add half a tablespoon of sauerkraut to each one.

Place the chicken thighs on a chopping board and cut them into big chunks or slices. Place on top of the sauerkraut, then spoon over a good zigzag of mayo, add the curry ketchup, chopped coriander and mint and finish with the lemon juice.

Roll up each wrap or naan as tightly as possible, wrapping it up in the paper or foil, then, using a sharp knife, cut in half, through the paper or foil, and turn each half outwards to show off the lovely colourful filling.

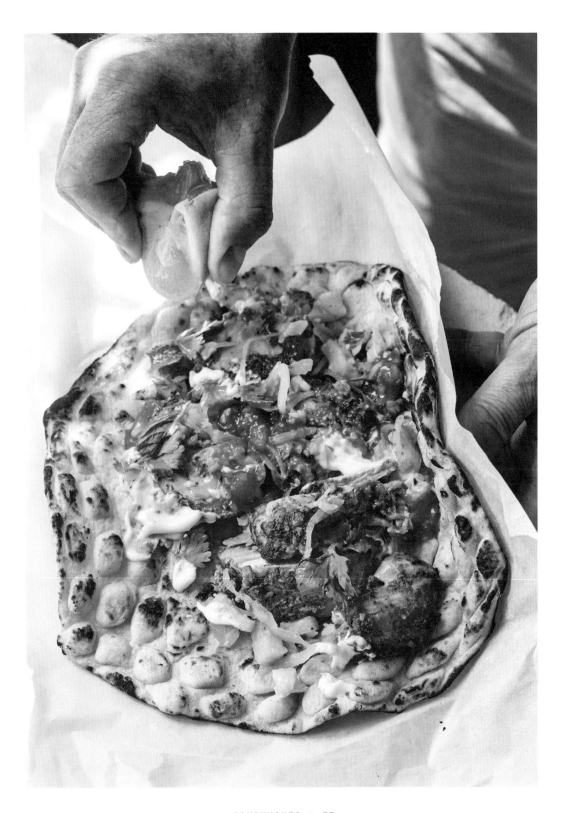

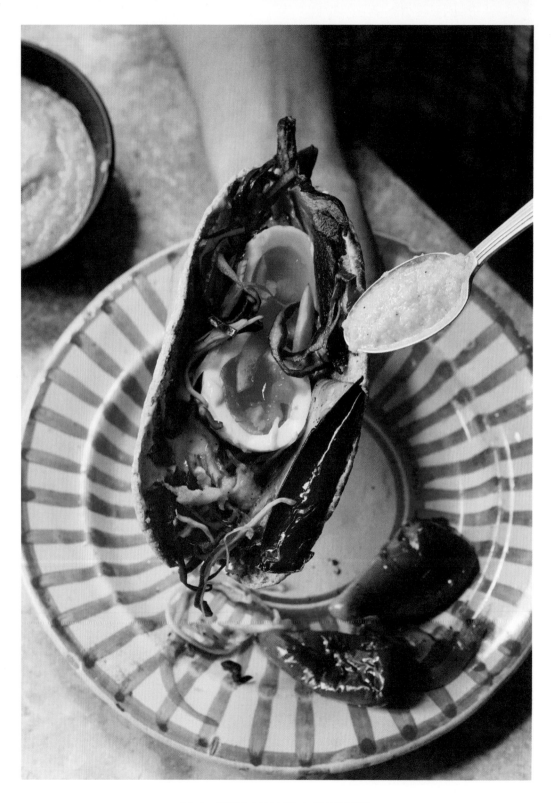

SABICH PITTA

I first tried this sandwich years ago, from a Tel Aviv street stall, then again years later at London's The Good Egg — it was so good, I wondered why I'd waited so long! The combination of aubergine slices, fried until chewy and sweet, and boiled eggs with creamy tahini and spicy amba sauce is truly magical. The addition of beetroot kimchi delivers the perfect tangy kick and great colour, and also offsets the richness, which is precisely what a good pickle should do. If preparing large batches of this, you can slice the aubergines thicker, arrange them in a single layer on a large baking tray, then season and drizzle with vegetable oil before roasting in an oven at 200°C/180°C fan (400°F), Gas Mark 6, for about 25 minutes, turning halfway through.

1 egg

3 tablespoons vegetable oil

1 aubergine, cut lengthways into slices about 5mm (¼ inch) thick

1 handful of finely shredded red cabbage

1 handful of finely shredded white cabbage

½ small onion, finely shredded

1 tablespoon olive oil

a squeeze of juice from ½ lemon

1 good-quality wholemeal or white pitta bread

1 heaped tablespoon Vadasz Super-Beet Kimchi or homemade Beetroot Kimchi (see page 25)

1 tablespoon Amba Sauce (see page 83)

salt and pepper

a few Mixed Chillies en Escabeche (see page 48), to serve

FOR THE TAHINI SAUCE

2 tablespoons tahini

½ garlic clove, crushed

juice of ½ lemon

2 tablespoons brine from Vadasz Garlic & Dill Pickles or brine from homemade Pickled Red Onions or Quick Cucumber Pickle (see pages 38 or 41)

1–2 tablespoons ice-cold water

First make the tahini sauce. Put the tahini, garlic, lemon juice and pickle brine in a small bowl and whisk together until combined, then whisk in the ice-cold water until smooth. Season to taste with salt and pepper.

Bring a small a saucepan of water to the boil, add the egg and boil for 7 minutes. Using a slotted spoon, transfer immediately to a bowl of cold water. When ready to use, shell and halve.

Heat a large heavy-based frying pan over a medium-high heat, then add the vegetable oil. Season the aubergine slices with salt and pepper, add to the hot pan — in batches if necessary — and fry for 1–2 minutes on each side until soft, well browned and crisp around the edges. Transfer to a plate lined with kitchen paper to absorb the excess oil.

While the aubergines are cooking or resting, put the cabbage, onion, olive oil and lemon juice in a mixing bowl, season generously with salt and pepper and mix well.

Toast your pitta bread in the toaster, then carefully slice into the top to open it up.

Holding the pitta bread in one hand, add the cabbage mixture, then the boiled egg halves, followed by the fried aubergine and the kimchi — you want the pitta to be overflowing, so don't hold back. Finish with a tablespoon of the tahini sauce, top with Chillies en Escabeche and a big spoonful of amba sauce.

Either wrap up the pitta in a square of food wrapping paper or foil to serve one, or cut in half to serve two as a snack, with plenty of kitchen paper!

EGG MAYONNAISE, PAPRIKA & PICKLE SANDWICH

My dad used to make this sandwich for picnics and packed lunches when we were kids. With that nostalgia in mind, the key to creating a memorable sandwich is to use the most appropriate bread to complement the filling which should be made with the best-quality ingredients. So an exemplary egg mayonnaise sandwich must have a soft, creamy egg mixture encased in a freshly baked baguette with softness at its heart, yet a crisp crust that gives easily when you bite into it and has that unique French bread flavour and aroma. The addition of a layer of pickles adds the perfect sweet-sour crunch to balance the richness of the egg. And the green peppers? Well, that's what Dad would use, and it wouldn't be the same without them!

4 eggs

1 heaped tablespoon good-quality mayonnaise

3 spring onions, fairly finely chopped

1 tablespoon finely diced green pepper

1 teaspoon English mustard

1 big pinch of paprika

1 long baguette, sliced in half lengthways and then into 3 portions

butter, for spreading

9–12 slices of Vadasz Garlic & Dill Pickles or homemade Quick Cucumber Pickle (see page 41), drained and patted dry with kitchen paper

salt and pepper

Bring a saucepan of water to the boil, add the eggs and boil for 10 minutes.

While the eggs are cooking, put the mayonnaise in a bowl with the spring onions, green pepper, mustard, paprika, some salt and plenty (and I mean plenty) of finely ground black pepper and mix well.

When the eggs are cooked, use a slotted spoon to transfer them to a bowl of cold water and leave to rest for 2 minutes.

Carefully shell the eggs, then add them to the mayonnaise mixture.

Using the edge of a tablespoon, chop the eggs roughly into quarters and then, focusing on the yolks, use the back of the spoon to mash them up and mix well — you want the yolks to be fully incorporated into the mayo but some of the whites to retain a bit of size.

Toast the baguette portions lightly and spread with butter, then divide the egg mayo mixture between the portions, spreading it on both the top and bottom pieces. Lay 3–4 pickle slices over each bottom piece and cover with the top pieces of baguette. Using a serrated knife, carefully cut each baguette portion in half to serve.

TUNA, AVOCADO & PICKLED FENNEL SANDWICH

There are so many great sandwich concepts, it was hard to choose what to include when putting this book together. Tuna mayo could be regarded as too everyday to make the cut, but this recipe breathes new life into the classic with the addition of pickled fennel. And if, like me, you're someone who loves that canned fish with chilli swimming around in the oil, then you'll really enjoy this recipe. Which reminds me, I have indeed made this with canned mackerel or sardines instead of tuna, and very suitable substitutes they are too.

300g (10½oz) good-quality canned tuna in sunflower oil (do not drain)

1 teaspoon small capers, drained

2 tablespoons mayonnaise

grated zest and juice of 1 lemon

1 ciabatta loaf

1 ripe avocado, peeled, stoned and sliced

1 tablespoon Pickled Fennel with Lemon (see page 44)

1 handful of flat leaf parsley, roughly chopped

1 pinch of Turkish chilli flakes or pul biber/Aleppo chilli flakes

salt and pepper

Put the tuna (with its oil), capers, mayo, lemon zest and a pinch of salt and pepper into a bowl and mix well until creamy but retaining some texture.

Slice the ciabatta in half lengthways and generously spread both halves with the tuna mixture.

Add the avocado to one ciabatta half, then sprinkle over the pickled fennel, lemon juice, parsley and chilli flakes. Top with the other ciabatta half.

Wrap tightly in greaseproof paper or foil and cut in half to reveal the lovely filling.

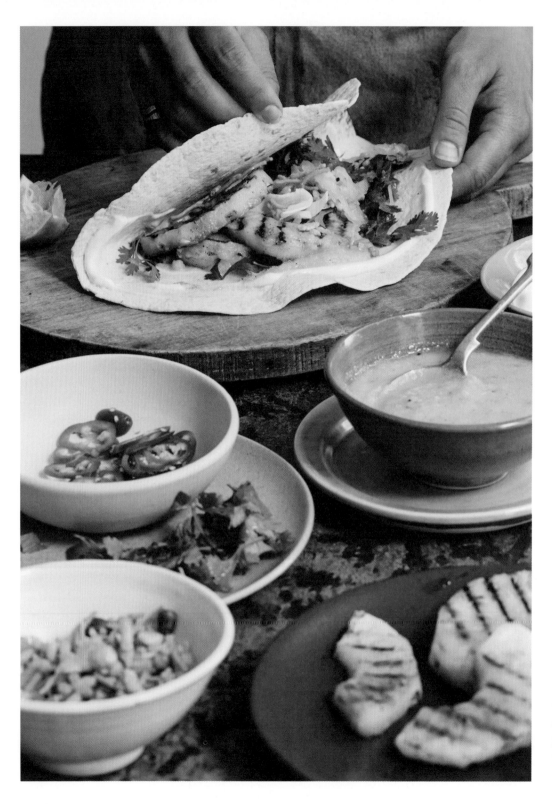

GRILLED PINEAPPLE, COCONUT & AMBA WRAP

Modern chefs routinely put vegetables at the heart of their dishes to create menus that are all the more diverse, dynamic and creative. Warm and sweet, juicy and savoury, I've used pineapple here as the 'meat' in my sandwich with glorious results! The amba sauce is extremely versatile, really good in a cheese sandwich or as a base for coronation chicken (or prawns) and features in the wonderful Sabich Pitta on page 79.

2 slices of fresh pineapple, about 2cm (¾ inch) thick, peeled and cored

vegetable oil

1 large flour tortilla, wrap, roti or flatbread

1 tablespoon vegan coconut yogurt

2 tablespoons Vadasz Pineapple & Turmeric Sauerkraut or homemade Curried Kraut (see page 27)

1 big pinch of toasted coconut chips

2 tablespoons Bombay mix, plus extra to garnish

1 handful of roughly chopped coriander, plus extra to garnish

1 handful of roughly chopped mint, plus extra to garnish

1 red or green chilli, very thinly sliced

salt and pepper

1 lime wedge, to serve

FOR THE AMBA SAUCE
(makes 180g/6¼oz)

100g (3½oz) Vadasz Pineapple & Turmeric Sauerkraut or homemade Curried Kraut (see page 27), plus 3 tablespoons of the brine

1 teaspoon English mustard

80ml (2¾fl oz) vegetable oil

First make the amba sauce. Put all the ingredients, except the oil, in a food processor or blender and blend as smooth as you can get it. With the machine running, drizzle in the vegetable oil slowly until emulsified. Season to taste with salt and pepper. (Any leftover sauce can be stored in the fridge for up to 5 days.)

Heat a heavy-based frying pan over a medium-high heat. While the pan is heating up, rub the pineapple with a drop of vegetable oil and season generously with salt and pepper.

When the pan is good and hot, slide in the pineapple slices and cook for about 5 minutes on each side – you want them slightly charred, as if barbecued. Transfer to a plate.

Working quickly, add your wrap of choice to the pan over a gentle heat to warm through while spreading the yogurt across the surface, then place the charred pineapple slices over one side of the wrap, and the remaining ingredients on top. Fold over the other half of the wrap to cover the filling.

Slide the folded wrap onto a chopping board and cut into 3 or 4 triangles. Pile on top of each other on 1 or 2 plates and add some more amba sauce and the extra herbs and Bombay mix to garnish. Serve with the lime wedge on the side for squeezing over.

TOFU BANH MI WITH DO CHUA PICKLES & KIMCHI

A legacy sandwich that often contains French components but is one hundred per cent Vietnamese, this is in my view one of the world's greatest, featuring one of the best pickles you can get. Here I'm using kimchi as well as the do chua pickles, which adds another layer of flavour and texture to a sandwich that is already abundant in both.

280g (10oz) block of firm tofu, patted dry with kitchen paper and cut into 3 or 4 thick slices

3 tablespoons vegetable oil

2 tablespoons cornflour

1 small or ⅓ of a large baguette

a good squirt of mayonnaise

2 tablespoons Vadasz Kimchi or homemade Kimchi (see page 24)

1 handful of Do Chua Vietnamese Pickles (see page 42)

1 handful of mint leaves

1 handful of coriander leaves

2 spring onions, sliced

6 slices of cucumber, cut at an angle

1 handful of roasted, salted peanuts, lightly crushed

a good drizzle of sriracha, if you like

FOR THE TOFU MARINADE

1 tablespoon sesame oil

½ tablespoon soy sauce

1 garlic clove, finely chopped

1 tablespoon rice wine or apple cider vinegar

salt and pepper

First make the tofu marinade. Put all the ingredients in a bowl and stir together well. Add the tofu slices, turning gently to coat them, then let them sit in their sweet/savoury bath for a few minutes.

Heat the vegetable oil in a heavy-based frying pan over a medium-high heat. While it's heating up, add the cornflour to a separate bowl and season with salt and pepper. Now add the tofu slices, one by one, gently tossing to coat them all over. Set aside the leftover marinade.

Carefully place the floured tofu in the hot pan and fry for about 2 minutes on each side, until crisp and golden. Transfer to a plate lined with kitchen paper to absorb the excess oil.

While the tofu is cooking and draining, slice the baguette open lengthways, then tear out any doughy bread inside, to avoid a soggy result. Squirt the mayo inside, then spoon in the kimchi.

Add the tofu, overlapping the slices along the length of the baguette. Now add the do chua pickles, the herbs, spring onions, cucumber and peanuts. Finish with the sriracha (if using) and a drizzle of the leftover tofu marinade.

To serve, lift the sandwich on to a sheet of foil, wrap it up snugly, then slice it in half to reveal the colourful layers inside. Remember, a tight wrap will ensure most of this wonderful sandwich ends up where it belongs — in your mouth and not down your front!

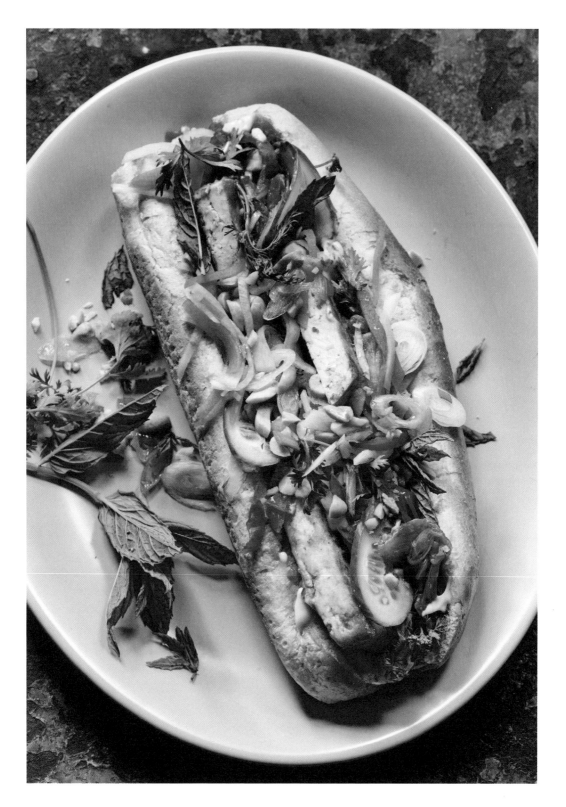

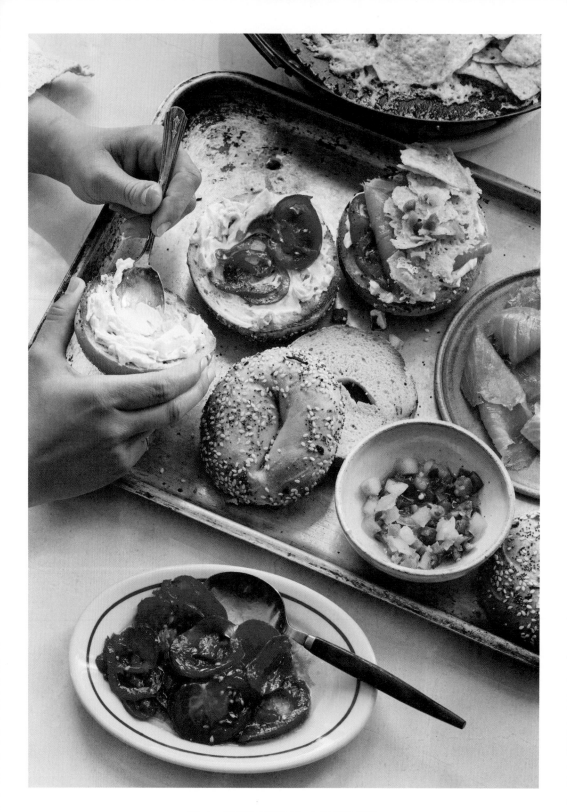

TOTOPOS CRUNCH, CREAM CHEESE & JALAPEÑO BAGELS

If I had to choose one bread to eat everything in, it would probably be a bagel; soft, chewy, but substantial enough to meet almost any textural challenge, and this twist on a traditional smoked salmon and cream cheese combo could be a contender for my default bagel filling. The jalapeño relish, mellowed by the creamy cheese, provides a comfy bed for the crunchy yet giving layer of cheesy grilled corn chips, with a layer of fresh tomato salsa and succulent smoked salmon sealing the deal. But feel free to use another protein of your choice: thinly sliced cooked turkey, chicken or chorizo, tuna mayo, or go vegan or veggie with avocado, shredded slaw or baby spinach.

165g (5¾oz) cream cheese

1 heaped tablespoon Vadasz Jalapeño Relish or homemade Jalapeño Relish (see page 49), drained, plus a little extra to finish

1 teaspoon vegetable oil

3 handfuls of grated Cheddar cheese

3 handfuls of plain corn chips

3 seeded, plain or everything bagels

100g (3½oz) good-quality smoked salmon

FOR THE SALSA

2 tomatoes

1 pinch each of salt and pepper

½ tablespoon olive oil

First make the simple salsa. Cut the tomatoes into wafer-thin slices and put in a bowl. Season with the salt and pepper and drizzle with the olive oil. Set aside until needed.

Whip the cream cheese with the heaped tablespoon of the jalapeño relish in a mixing bowl and set aside until needed.

Heat a large, heavy-based frying pan over a low to medium heat and add the vegetable oil, rotating and tilting the pan to cover the base. Sprinkle with the cheese, and as it begins to melt, scatter the corn chips over the top. Then, using a wide metal spatula, gently crush the chips down so that they flatten and merge with the melting cheese.

Leave the cheese to continue melting and cooking while you slice the bagels in half and toast lightly. Once the cheese has melted fully and is browning and crisping around the edge, take the pan off the heat.

Spread both halves of the bagels with the cream cheese mixture, then add a spoonful of the tomato salsa to the top halves and fold the smoked salmon on to the bottom halves.

Using the spatula, cut the cheesy corn chips into thirds and shovel each third on the smoked salmon halves — a nachos 'overhang' is a worthy goal here! Top with extra jalapeño relish.

Flip the salsa-covered top halves over on to the nacho-covered bottom halves. Slide each filled bagel on to a piece of greaseproof paper or foil big enough to accommodate your creation. Wrap tightly and slice in half to expose the beautiful layers inside, or just keep them whole. To my mind they always eat better from the paper or foil — less messy too!

DOUBLE PICKLE CHEESEBURGER

Trying to recreate the best burger you've ever had is a continual work in progress; ever evolving, always room for improvement. So this is a challenge for me and for you too. I've eaten many burgers in my life, some bad, some good and some very good indeed. This is my latest attempt using great beef (ideally formed from the best aged beef from your local butcher, or similar quality beef burgers from a really good retailer), classic American cheese and grilled onions, enhanced and 'Vadaszled' by pickles! My condiment preference, in addition to the pickles and grilled onions, is just really good hot mustard. But don't let me hold you back — add ketchup and/or mayo too if you want.

2 good-quality burger buns

soft butter, for spreading

2 x 170g (6oz) beef patties, removed from the fridge 20 minutes before cooking them

4 slices of American cheese

2 tablespoons Vadasz Red Onion Pickles or homemade Pickled Red Onions (see page 38), plus 2 tablespoons of the brine

2 thick slices from the middle of a large onion, around 1cm (½ inch) each (to match the dimensions of your burgers

2 teaspoons good English or Dijon mustard

8 slices of Vadasz Garlic & Dill Pickles or Quick Cucumber Pickle (see page 41)

a squirt of mayonnaise (optional)

a squirt of tomato ketchup (optional)

salt and pepper

fries, to serve

Heat a large heavy-based frying pan over a medium-high heat.

Slice your buns in half and butter the cut sides well, right to the edge. Add them, cut side down, to the hot pan and toast for just a minute or so to seal them. Remove from the pan and set aside.

Place the patties gently in the hot pan, season well with salt and pepper (if not already added) and cook for 4 minutes, or until the undersides are well seared with a deep brown crust. Flip them over and top each patty with 2 cheese slices — the second slice offset from the first to resemble an 8-pointed star so that you'll get a good all-round melt.

Have a pan lid at the ready, then add the red onion pickles to the patties, followed by the brine. As this hits the pan and starts to sizzle, cover immediately with the lid to harness the steam, which will melt the cheese in about 20 seconds. Remove the lid and place the top halves of the buns on the burgers, still in the pan. Let them sizzle away for about 4 minutes more (if you prefer grilled onion in your burger, add the onion rings to the pan too and turn once or twice until the caramelized colour you want).

Smear the bottom halves of the buns with the mustard, add the cucumber pickles, and an onion ring, followed by a squirt of mayo and ketchup, if using.

Using a firm spatula, shovel the bun-topped burgers out of the pan and onto the fully dressed bottom halves of the buns. Serve with fries and a mile or two of kitchen paper.

Note: The cooking times above are for a medium-cooked burger. For medium-well done, lower the heat and cook for a further 1–2 minutes on each side.

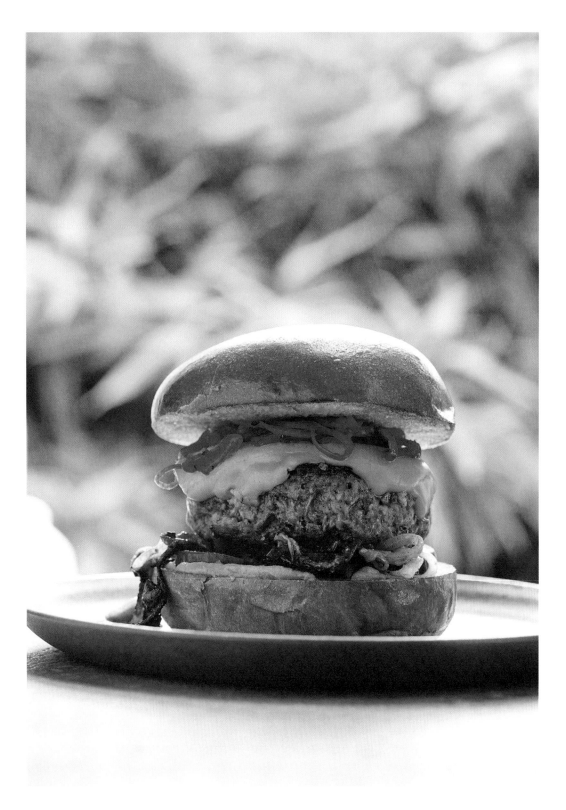

SOUPS & SALADS

CAULIFLOWER & LENTIL SOUP WITH CURRIED PINEAPPLE SAUERKRAUT

This is the kind of soup that fills the kitchen with welcoming curry aromas on a cold winter's night. At its heart are the warm, deep tangy flavours that emerge from the pineapple and turmeric sauerkraut, adding a fermented punch to the earthy lentils and cauliflower.

1 small or ½ large cauliflower

olive oil

1 onion, sliced

1 small carrot, diced

1 bay leaf

200g (7oz) Vadasz Pineapple & Turmeric Sauerkraut or homemade Curried Kraut (see page 27), plus extra to serve

1 teaspoon brown miso paste

300g (10½oz) dried red split lentils, well rinsed and drained

900ml (1½ pints) water

juice of ½ lemon

salt and pepper

FOR THE SPICY OIL

4 tablespoons olive oil

1 red chilli, finely sliced

3 garlic cloves, finely chopped

1 thumb-sized piece of fresh root ginger, scrubbed and grated

a few spring onions, finely sliced

2 teaspoons garam masala

TO SERVE

natural yogurt, or coconut yogurt for a vegan option

handful of coriander, leaves picked

To prepare your cauliflower, trim the tough base of the stem and remove any tough outer leaves, then cut off the remaining leaves and stem and roughly chop. Hold the cauliflower, stem end down, on a chopping board, and cut into slices 2cm (¾ inch) thick, reserving any remaining florets.

Heat a drizzle of olive oil in a wide saucepan over a medium heat. Add the cauliflower slices, along with the chopped stem, leaves and florets, and sear for 6–8 minutes, until well coloured on both sides (the leaves will take less time). You might have to do this in batches, depending on the size of your pan. Transfer to a dish and set aside.

Add more olive oil to the pan and gently fry the onion and carrot with the bay leaf and a pinch of salt for 2–3 minutes. Add the sauerkraut and stir-fry for a few minutes, until the kraut dries out and colours slightly. Stir through the miso.

Add the rinsed lentils and seared cauliflower to the pan, season well with salt and pepper and pour over the measured water (you might have to add more, depending on the size of your cauliflower – you want all the ingredients to be well covered by water to help them cook). Bring to the boil, then reduce the heat, cover the pan and simmer for 20–25 minutes, or until the cauliflower and lentils are tender but not mushy.

While the soup is simmering, prepare the spicy oil. Heat the olive oil in a frying pan over a medium heat, add the chilli, garlic, ginger and spring onions and cook for about 3 minutes, until well coloured, stirring in the garam masala at the end.

When the cauliflower and lentils are ready, remove the bay leaf and take the pan off the heat, then tilt it slightly and use a stick blender to blitz your soup just a little until you have a suitably rustic soup texture – you want to keep the cauliflower chunky.

Mix the spicy oil into the soup, stir through the lemon juice and season to taste with salt and pepper.

Ladle the soup into big bowls and top with more of the sauerkraut, a blob of dairy or coconut yogurt and some coriander leaves.

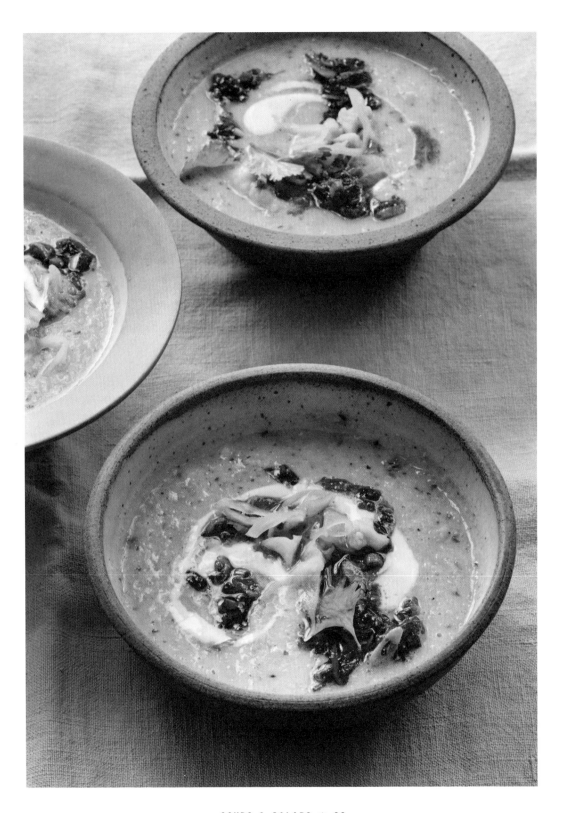

DAD'S HANGOVER SOUP

While selling my pickles at the wonderful Brockley Market in southeast London on Saturday mornings, I was often asked for a shot of pickle brine by a small group of discerning customers, all of Eastern European heritage. I mentioned this and the fact that, according to them, it was a renowned cure for even the most severe hangovers, to my dad, and he confirmed that it was a common cure for alcohol over-indulgence in Hungary. He also told me about hangover or pickle soup, which apparently had the same therapeutic effect — the magical forces of fermented cabbage! It may indeed be beneficial in that way, but it's also an all-round, feel-good, nourishing soup.

For a vegan version, omit the sausage and add a touch more paprika or a tiny pinch of smoked paprika, and instead of adding the soured cream and flour, use a stick blender to blend the soup a little to thicken it slightly.

1 tablespoon vegetable oil

1 onion, diced

1 small carrot, diced

½ celery stick, diced

1 bay leaf

100g (3½oz) gyulai sausage (Hungarian smoked pork sausage) or chorizo sausage, quartered lengthways, then sliced

½ tablespoon paprika

400g (14oz) Vadasz Garlic & Dill Sauerkraut or homemade Sauerkraut with Garlic & Dill (see page 26)

1 litre (1¾ pints) water

2 tablespoons soured cream, plus extra to garnish

1 tablespoon plain flour

1 pinch of sugar

salt and pepper

1 handful of fresh dill, chopped, to garnish

fresh bread, to serve

Heat the vegetable oil in a large saucepan over a medium heat, add the onion, carrot and celery and sweat for about 3 minutes, until softened.

Throw in the bay leaf, the sausage and paprika and stir well for a minute or so.

Add the sauerkraut, pour in the measured water and stir well, then bring to a simmer and simmer for 10 minutes or so.

While the soup is simmering, mix the soured cream and flour together in the empty sauerkraut pot or a small bowl.

Add the soured cream mixture to the pan and stir briskly until it's completely combined. Continue to stir gently as the soup returns to a simmer, and simmer for another 5 minutes to cook out the flour properly.

Taste the soup for seasoning, adding more salt if needed, along with the touch of sugar just to balance out the flavour.

Ladle the soup into large bowls and garnish with an extra dollop of soured cream and the chopped dill. Serve with good fresh bread.

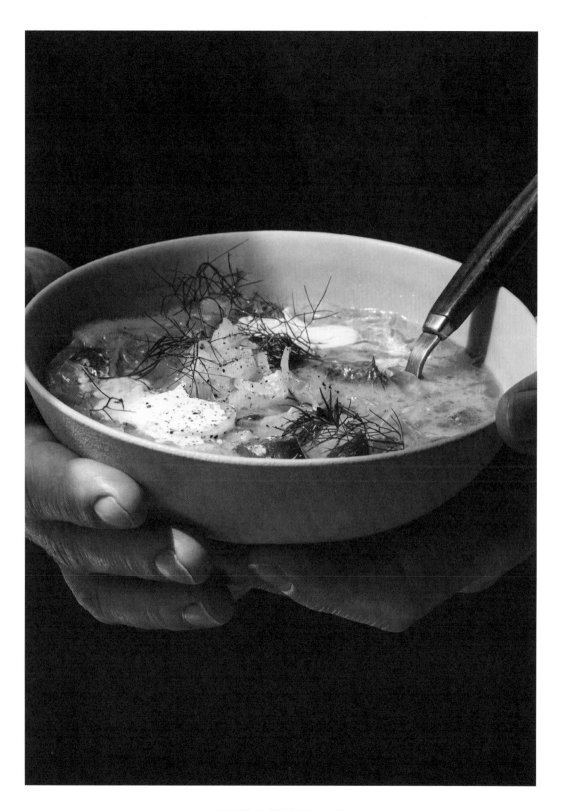

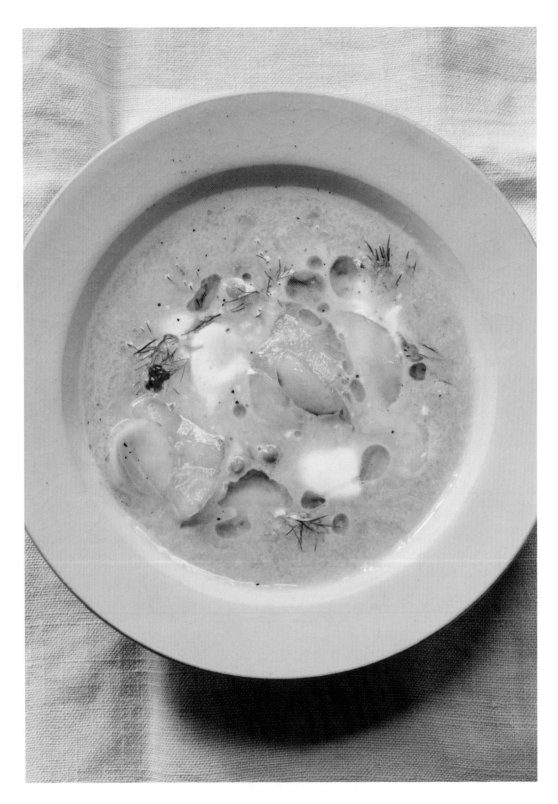

PEA & PICKLE SOUP

Like all decent cooks, I find the best things I make tend to be unplanned, impulsive and intuitive. This soup recipe was created as a result of me twisting my ankle and the need to reduce the swelling, which I did by applying a bag of frozen peas wrapped in a tea towel. It was a blessing that, by dinnertime, the peas were too defrosted to return to the freezer. Result: this simple, super-quick and dellcious soup! If you should have any leftovers, just reheat in a pan to reduce the liquid until you have a nice thick pea stew, which when spooned over a piece of heavily buttered crusty toast and dusted well with finely grated Parmesan cheese is as good, if not better than, the soup. It's great as a pasta sauce too.

1 tablespoon olive oil, plus an extra swirl to serve

1 small onion, finely chopped

1 small piece of celery, chopped

1 bay leaf

300g (10½oz) frozen peas

2 heaped tablespoons Vadasz Garlic & Dill Sauerkraut or homemade Sauerkraut with Garlic & Dill (see page 26), plus 1 forkful to serve, and 2–3 tablespoons of the brine

500ml (18fl oz) just-boiled water

a blob of butter

salt and pepper

TO SERVE

1 tablespoon soured cream

a few big pinches of chopped dill

a few slices of Vadasz Garlic & Dill Pickles or homemade Quick Cucumber Pickle (see page 41), chopped

Heat the olive oil in a medium-sized saucepan over a medium heat, add the onion, celery and bay leaf and sweat for just a minute or so. Stir in the peas and sauerkraut and season with salt and plenty of pepper. Pour the measured boiling water into the pan and stir well. Cover and simmer for 3–4 minutes, until the peas begin to change colour but not entirely — you want a fresh-tasting soup.

Add the butter and sauerkraut brine, then take the pan off the heat, tilt it slightly and use a stick blender to blitz the soup a little, but not too much, as you want to retain some of that pea texture.

Taste the soup for seasoning, adding extra salt and pepper if needed, then serve in bowls topped with the soured cream, dill, chopped pickles, extra kraut, a few drops of olive oil and a good twist of black pepper.

KALE, APRICOT & CURRIED KRAUT SALAD WITH ALMONDS & FETA

This recipe demonstrates so well how the sunny flavours and colour of Vadasz Pineapple & Turmeric Sauerkraut or your own homemade version can brighten up your salads and enliven your greens. Try using fresh pineapple or any other really sweet fruit instead of the soaked dried apricots, to balance the tang of the kraut.

½ tablespoon clear honey

4 tablespoons water

130g (4½oz) natural (unsulphured) dried apricots

125g (4¼oz) whole skin-on almonds

200g (7oz) cavolo nero or kale, stems trimmed and shredded, reserving 1 big handful for the dressing

2 garlic cloves, peeled

5 tablespoons extra virgin olive oil

juice of ½ lime, plus 1 lime, halved, for squeezing over

200g (7oz) Vadasz Pineapple & Turmeric Sauerkraut or homemade Curried Kraut (see page 27), plus 3 tablespoons of the brine for the dressing

100g (3½oz) feta cheese

salt and pepper

1 big handful of coriander, roughly chopped, to serve

Put the honey and water in a small bowl and mix well. Submerge the apricots in the honey solution and leave to soak for at least 20 minutes.

While the apricots are soaking, toast the almonds in a dry frying pan over a low heat for a few minutes, until their skins darken, tossing frequently to achieve an even colour. Take the pan off the heat and, as they cool, their crunchiness will develop.

Once cooled, add the almonds to a food processor and pulse just for a few seconds to break them up. Tip on to a plate and set aside. There's no need to wash out the food processor bowl, as you'll need it to make the dressing.

Once the apricots have finished soaking, make the dressing. Drain the honey solution into a food processor bowl and add 4 of the apricots setting the rest aside. Add the reserved cavolo nero or kale, sauerkraut brine, garlic cloves, olive oil and lime juice to the processor bowl. Blend until you have a smooth, thickened consistency. Season to taste with salt and pepper and set aside.

Slice the remaining soaked apricots into strips, add to a big salad bowl with the remaining shredded cavolo nero or kale and the sauerkraut and mix well. Add the almonds and the feta, crumbling the cheese into small pieces as you drop it in. Pour over the dressing and toss well.

To serve, pile up generously in wide salad bowls and top with the chopped coriander and lime halves for squeezing over.

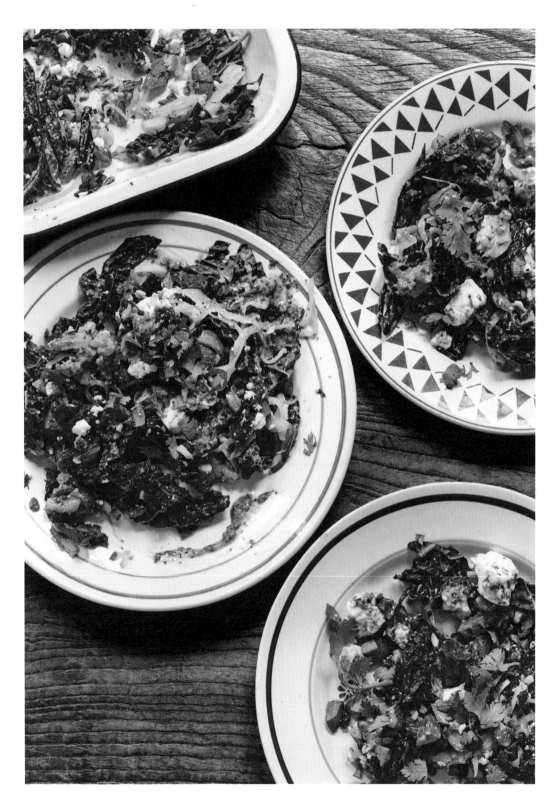

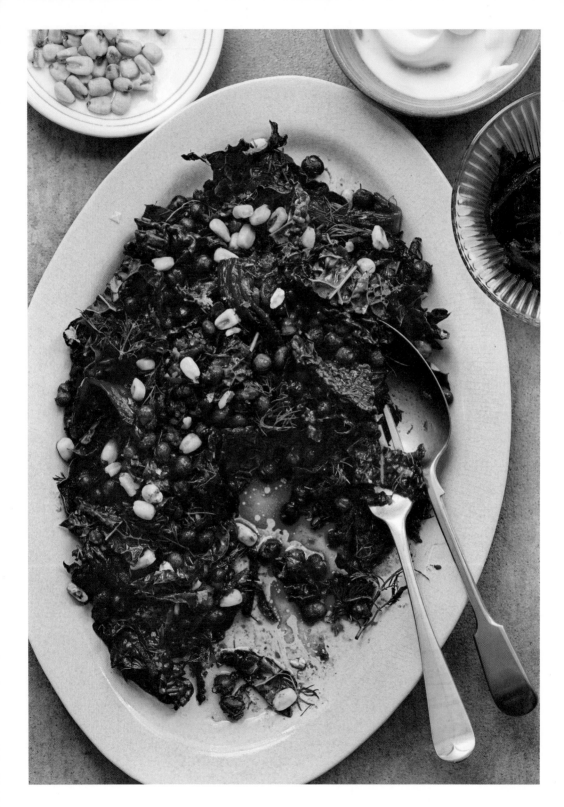

CARLIN PEAS, CAVOLO NERO & BEETROOT KIMCHI WITH DILL

This is a one-bowl salad and is ready in minutes — happy days! Carlin peas are similar to chickpeas but have a unique, earthy, nutty taste and are the star here, especially when matched with the Super-Beet Kimchi and some citrus zest. I've also used the full-flavoured liquid (aquafaba) they are canned in to embolden and enhance the dressing. But if you can't get Carlin peas, it's also delicious with chickpeas. If you have any leftovers, mix into a batch of cold cooked brown rice for a great work lunch pot (see page 113).

2 x 400g (14oz) cans Carlin peas or chickpeas, drained, reserving 3 tablespoons of their liquid

100g (3½oz) cavolo nero, stems trimmed and roughly chopped

200g (7oz) Vadasz Super-Beet Kimchi or homemade Beetroot Kimchi (see page 25), plus extra to serve

grated zest and juice of ½ lemon

grated zest of ¼ orange

juice of ½ orange

1 bunch of dill, roughly chopped

4 tablespoons olive oil, plus extra to serve

salt and pepper

TO SERVE

4–5 tablespoons coconut yogurt

roasted chickpeas, corn kernels or peanuts

Put the Carlin peas or chickpeas and their liquid in a big mixing bowl along with the cavolo nero, beetroot kimchi, lemon and orange zest and juice, dill and olive oil. Season with salt and pepper.

Using a spoon in each hand, toss everything together. Taste again for salt and pepper before piling into big salad bowls. Top each with a tablespoon of coconut yogurt, a forkful of extra beetroot kimchi, the roasted chickpeas, corn or peanuts for crunch, and a big swirl of olive oil.

GRILLED PINEAPPLE & BROCCOLI SALAD

It's Monday night and I'm craving something fairly simple and freshly cooked.
A brief forage in the fridge and I find half a pineapple, a block of feta, some
broccoli and spinach, a jar of roasted peppers and a pot of red onion pickles.
The resulting recipe is layers of sweet on sweet, well balanced by the acidity
of the feta and pickles. A good night's work indeed.

1 fresh pineapple – you will use only ½, so keep the remainder for another use

olive oil

1 small or ½ large head of broccoli

1 garlic clove, lightly crushed but left intact

1 splash of brine from the Vadasz Red Onion Fresh Pickles or homemade Pickled Red Onions (see page 38) – see 'To Serve' below – or water

about 450g (1lb) roasted red peppers from a jar

240g (8½oz) baby spinach

salt and pepper

FOR THE DRESSING

2 tablespoons olive oil

1 tablespoon soy sauce

1 splash of brine from the Vadasz Red Onion Fresh Pickles or homemade Pickled Red Onions (see page 38)

1 garlic clove, chopped

1 thumb-sized piece of fresh root ginger, scrubbed and cut into matchsticks

TO SERVE

3 big pinches of Vadasz Red Onion Pickles or homemade Pickled Red Onions (see page 38)

3 big pinches of crumbled feta cheese

Peel the whole pineapple and, holding it upright, cut 3 slices lengthways, including the core, about 1–2cm (½–¾ inch) thick. Season them well with a little salt and plenty of pepper, and drizzle with olive oil.

Slice the head of broccoli from top to bottom in the same way and to the same thickness as the pineapple, and again season with salt and pepper and drizzle with olive oil.

Heat a large, heavy griddle pan over a medium heat, and when hot, carefully add the pineapple slices – in batches if necessary – along with the garlic clove and cook for about 3 minutes on each side or until well grilled and browned. Transfer to a plate, cover loosely with foil and set aside to rest.

Add the broccoli to the hot griddle pan and again cook for a few minutes on each side until nicely browned. Pour in the pickle brine or water and cook until evaporated – this will help to steam your broccoli. Transfer to the plate with the pineapple and cover loosely with the foil.

While the pineapple and broccoli are cooking, make the dressing. Put all the ingredients in a bowl and whisk together, then set aside.

Now make a simple salsa: remove the peppers from the jar, dangle over a colander over a bowl and force the brine out between your finger and thumb until well drained. Place the squeezed peppers into a food processor or blender and blend until smooth. Season to taste with salt and pepper, then set aside until needed. Both this salsa and the dressing can be made ahead of time if you prefer.

Once the broccoli comes out of the pan, add the baby spinach – in batches if necessary – with a pinch of salt and pepper and stir-fry for 30 seconds or so, just until it wilts slightly.

To serve, spoon the red pepper salsa into the centre of 3 serving plates, then use the back of the spoon to spread it out. Pile up some of the spinach and add a slice of the pineapple and broccoli. Arrange a big pile of red onion pickles over the broccoli and spoon the dressing all ove. Finish off with the feta cheese, generously sprinkled like snow across the beautiful yellow, red and green landscape.

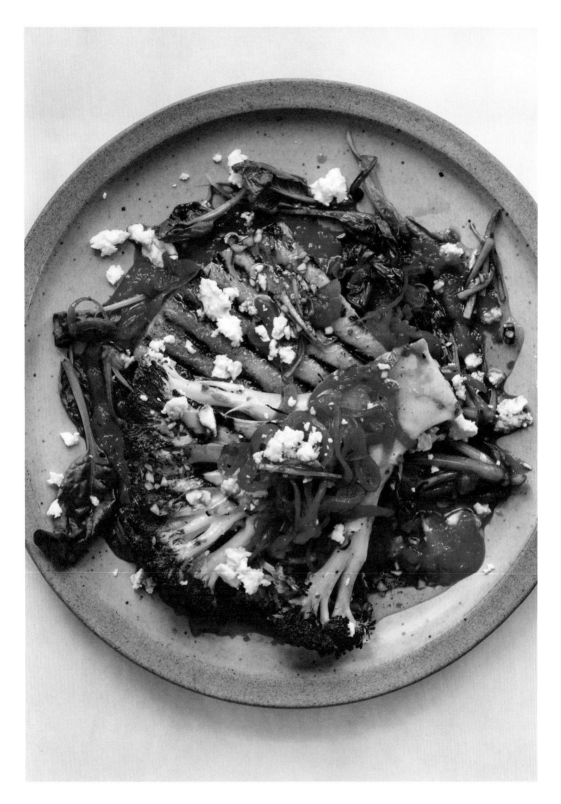

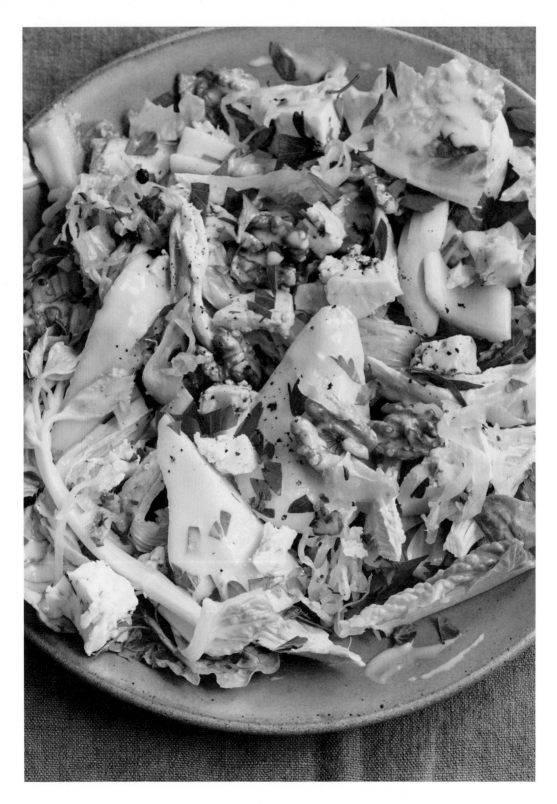

CHICKEN SALAD WITH PEARS, BLUE CHEESE & FERMENTED CELERY

As American classics go, a Waldorf salad done well is a joy, but is improved considerably, in my opinion, with the addition of a few clumps of strong blue cheese along with familiar pear-ings and the gentle jolt of fermented acidity. We often have this on a Monday, or variations of it, making good use of Sunday's roast. You can, of course, lose the chicken altogether if you want a veggie version.

½ roast chicken, meat picked (about 170–200g 6–7oz)

2 sticks of Fermented Celery (see page 32) or fresh celery, cut into 2cm (¾ inch) pieces, plus the leaves to garnish

50g (1¾oz) walnut halves

1 large firm but sweet pear, peeled if liked, then quartered, cored and cut into big chunks

½ large Romaine lettuce, quartered lengthways and torn into big pieces

40g (1½oz) Stichelton cheese or other creamy blue cheese, broken into pieces, plus an extra 20g (1¾oz) to serve

2 tablespoons Vadasz Garlic & Dill Sauerkraut or homemade Sauerkraut with Garlic & Dill (see page 26)

1 handful of flat leaf parsley, chopped, to garnish

FOR THE DRESSING

1 tablespoon mayonnaise

1 tablespoon single cream

2 teaspoons apple cider vinegar

1 teaspoon English mustard

4 tablespoons extra virgin olive oil

salt and pepper

Put all the salad ingredients in a large bowl but don't mix anything yet.

To make the dressing, put the mayo, cream, vinegar and mustard in a small bowl and then, while whisking vigorously, drizzle in the olive oil until it's thick and creamy. Taste and season with salt and pepper.

Pour the dressing over the salad and very gently mix together with your hands.

To serve, arrange the salad on plates, garnishing with the extra cheese, the celery leaves and chopped parsley, finishing with a twist of black pepper.

SMOKED MACKEREL, POTATOES & ASPARAGUS WITH PICKLED ONIONS

I love cold fish or meat with warm potatoes — be they mashed, fried or, as in this case, boiled with carrots. The method here is to dress the potatoes and carrots while they are still warm from cooking so that they absorb everything you throw at them — butter, mustard, parsley and crushed caraway. As they cool down, and by the time you serve them, they will have become perfectly seasoned and balanced, enriched and elevated. Along with dainty asparagus spears and smoky, oily fish, the stage is then set for some pirouetting, pretty pink pickled onions to complete the choreography.

1kg (2lb 4oz) new potatoes, scrubbed

2 large carrots, each cut into 4 chunks

2 eggs

1 bunch of thin asparagus spears, well washed

a big blob of butter

1 heaped teaspoon Dijon mustard

1 big handful of flat leaf parsley, chopped

1 pinch of caraway seeds, crushed

4 smoked mackerel fillets, any stray bones removed

salt and pepper

TO SERVE

1½ tablespoons capers, drained

200g (7oz) Vadasz Red Onion Pickles or homemade Pickled Red Onions (see page 38)

a big swirl of extra virgin olive oil

1 tablespoon mayonnaise

1 pinch of paprika

Bring a large saucepan of salted water to the boil, add the potatoes and carrots and boil for 15 minutes or until firm but fully cooked through when prodded with a fork.

When the potatoes and carrots have been cooking for 9 minutes, add the eggs to the same pan and, once the water has returned to a rolling boil, set a timer for 3 minutes.

After the 3 minutes is up, add the asparagus, then again set the timer for 3 minutes (but bear in mind that the asparagus might take more or less time depending on thickness).

When the eggs have cooked for 6 minutes in total, use a slotted spoon to transfer them to a bowl of cold water; when the asparagus is cooked, transfer it to a separate bowl. When the eggs are cool enough to handle, shell them and set aside until needed.

When the potatoes and carrots are ready, drain and let them steam-dry in the colander for a couple of minutes. Tumble them into a big mixing bowl and add the other ingredients, but don't mix yet. Add the butter first, followed by the mustard, most of the parsley (reserving some to garnish) and then the caraway seeds.

Add the asparagus, season with salt and pepper and then, using a spoon in each hand, gently bring everything together. If the potatoes are big, halve them with the side of your spoon as you mix, but don't overdo it — you want broken potato boulders not mashed potatoes.

To serve, pile some of the potato mix to one side of each plate, followed by the mackerel fillet on the other side. Scatter over the capers, followed by a loose tower of red onion pickles. Finish with a big swirl of olive oil, the reserved parsley, a dollop of mayonnaise and a sprinkling of paprika.

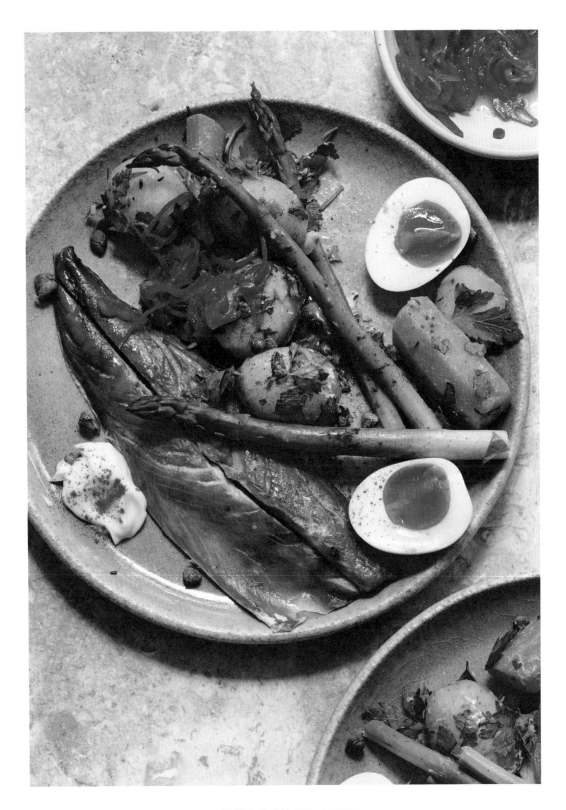

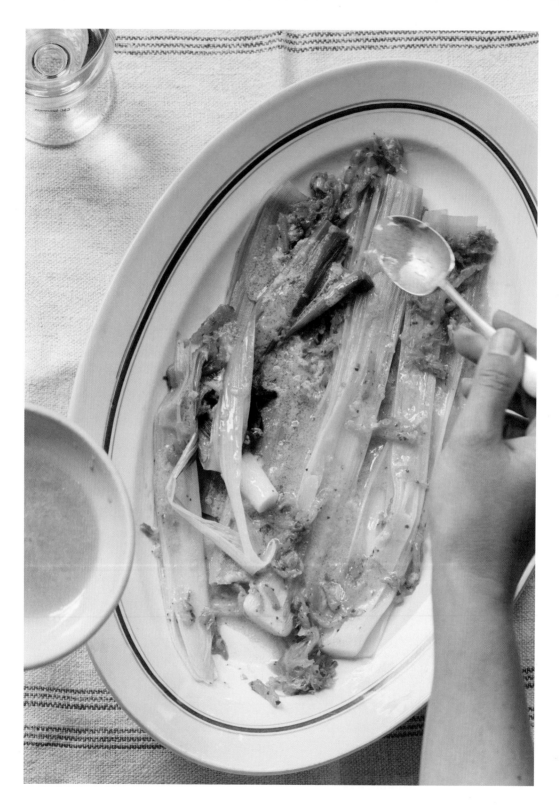

LEEKS WITH KIMCHI VINAIGRETTE

I'm a big fan of this classic dish, but I'd been planning to try it with kimchi
for ages, and when I finally got around to it, I wasn't disappointed.
Enlivening the soft, sweet fleshy leeks with the funk of kimchi is an
extremely worthwhile refinement. If you use baby leeks instead of
large ones, reduce the cooking time accordingly.

3 leeks, trimmed (remove outer layers and/or tough green ends), halved lengthways and rinsed of any dirt

1 tablespoon olive oil

1 tablespoon Vadasz Kimchi or homemade Kimchi (see page 24), plus 1 tablespoon of the brine for the vinaigrette

salt and pepper

FOR THE VINAIGRETTE

1 teaspoon Dijon mustard

1 tablespoon apple cider vinegar

1 garlic clove, crushed

3 tablespoons olive oil

Place your leeks with the residual water from rinsing them in a wide pan over a medium-low heat, along with the olive oil and kimchi. Season well with salt and pepper.

Cover the pan and cook the leeks gently for 10–15 minutes — you might need to add a drop of water if the pan dries out. Check their progress by prodding with a fork: they should be soft, with little or no resistance. Give them a little longer if needed.

While the leeks are cooking, make the vinaigrette. Put the mustard, kimchi brine, vinegar and garlic in a small bowl and mix well, then whisk in the olive oil with a fork. Season with a little salt and pepper.

Once the leeks are ready, leave to cool for 10–15 minutes before drenching with the vinaigrette.

TORTILLA SALAD WITH JALAPEÑO RELISH

Back in the early 1990s I worked in a Tex-Mex restaurant where this salad was served in a giant, deep-fried flour tortilla shaped like a bowl, the idea being that you ate the salad *and* the bowl, pools of deep-fryer fat and all! I've ditched the oily edible vessel and focused on creating a landscape of great flavour and texture: cheese, hot beans, corn chips and jalapeño relish all come together beautifully as you excavate through the layers. This is great served family-style in a large, shallow serving bowl as a centrepiece.

4 big handfuls of mixed salad – I use Little Gem lettuce, shredded red cabbage and sliced onions

4 handfuls of good-quality plain corn chips, crushed a little as they leave your hand

8 tablespoons warm Braised Beans (see page 124)

340g (12oz) can sweetcorn, drained

1 red pepper, cored, deseeded and diced or sliced

200g (7oz) feta cheese

4 tablespoons Vadasz Jalapeño Relish or homemade Jalapeño Relish (see page 49)

1 dollop of soured cream

1 handful of toasted corn kernels

1 handful of coriander, chopped

a swirl of olive oil

2 limes, quartered

Start to layer up the ingredients in a wide salad bowl. I like to do this in rough rows so that all the items are visible when finished. First cover the bottom of the bowl with the mixed salad, then add the corn chips, followed by the warm beans.

Add a pile of the sweetcorn and red pepper, then scatter over the feta, crumbling it as you go.

Finish with the jalapeño relish, soured cream, toasted corn kernels, chopped coriander and olive oil. Finish by squeezing the juice from the lime quarters over the salad – leaving the quarters on top gives the salad a good aroma from the lime zest.

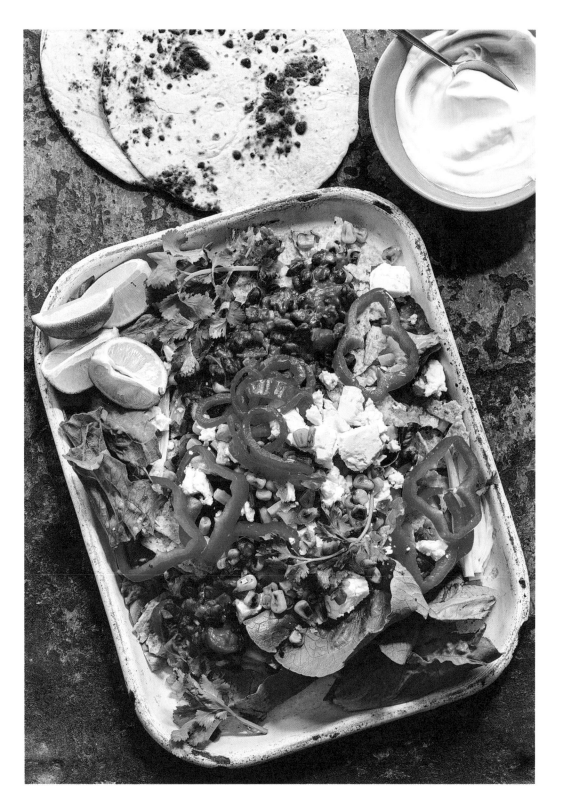

WARM CURRIED POTATO SALAD

Behold! A potato salad inspired by Bombay aloo! Seasoned with golden curry-flavoured sauerkraut, the warm potatoes engage with the spicy kraut to enliven the salad far more successfully than cold potatoes will. Great as a side with grilled meats, other small plates or mezze, or lovely as a meal on its own; brunch it up by adding soft-boiled or poached eggs and/or crispy bacon.

750g (1lb 10½oz) white potatoes, such as King Edward or Maris Piper

3 tablespoons vegetable oil

1 onion, sliced

4 tomatoes, quartered

3-4 tablespoons Vadasz Pineapple & Turmeric Sauerkraut or homemade Curried Kraut (see page 27), plus extra to serve

2 teaspoons garam masala

1 bay leaf

1 long green chilli, thinly sliced

100g (3½oz) frozen peas, defrosted

2 tablespoons mayonnaise

1 big handful of fresh coriander, chopped

salt and pepper

Peel and wash the potatoes, then halve (or quarter them if necessary) so that they are all roughly the same size. Place in a large pan of salted water, bring to the boil, then reduce the heat and simmer for around 15–20 minutes, until soft enough to break when prodded with a fork but still retain some texture.

While the potatoes are cooking, heat the vegetable oil in a large frying pan over a medium heat, then add the onion, tomatoes, sauerkraut, garam masala, the bay leaf and sliced chilli. Season with salt and pepper and stir-fry gently for about 10 minutes, until the onions have softened but are not too brown. Remove from the heat and set aside.

When the potatoes are cooked, drain, then allow to steam-dry for a minute or two.

Transfer the potatoes to a large mixing bowl along with the stir-fried ingredients, then add the peas and the mayonnaise and mix well.

Serve topped with some extra sauerkraut and a load of fresh coriander.

VADASZ POTTED LUNCHES

'Where's that small Tupperware container? You know the one!'

If I had a pound for every time I've heard this question in our house...
Enter, stage left, the joy of an empty Vadasz pot or similar, upcycled to
carry your lunch in.

Throughout this book I encourage you to use your brine, even the last few
drops, along with the remaining scraps of pickle, sauerkraut or kimchi — even
just a spoonful of the spicy debris can transform and add value to everything
you make. But when your pot is truly empty, it becomes the perfect vessel for
leftovers, sauces, dressings and lunch on the go.

Here's an example of what I put in my pots for lunch, whether I'm at the
office, travelling by train or going on a picnic, made from what you might
have in the fridge or store cupboard, packed the night before, left to chill
and ready to go. The trick is to layer purposefully and leave enough
headspace in order to be able to mix before forking it mouthwards.

The only issue — remembering to grab it as you dash out the door!

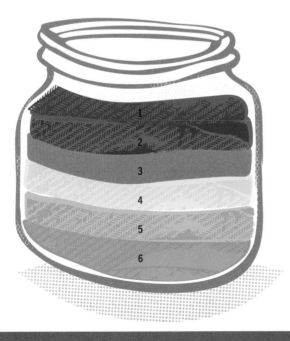

1. **TOPPINGS** — hot sauce, seeds, nuts

2. **PICKLES** — kimchi, sauerkraut, pickles, jalapeño relish

3. **SAUCES OR DIPS** — hummus, tzatziki

4. **VEGETABLES** — cooked broccoli or beetroot, raw green beans or grated carrots

5. **MEAT OR DAIRY PROTEIN** — cooked chicken, canned fish, boiled egg, hard or soft cheese

   OR

   VEGETABLE PROTEIN OR PULSES AND NUTS — canned black beans or lentils, roasted almonds, walnuts

6. **COOKED GRAINS OR CARBOHYDRATES** — cold cooked brown rice or barley

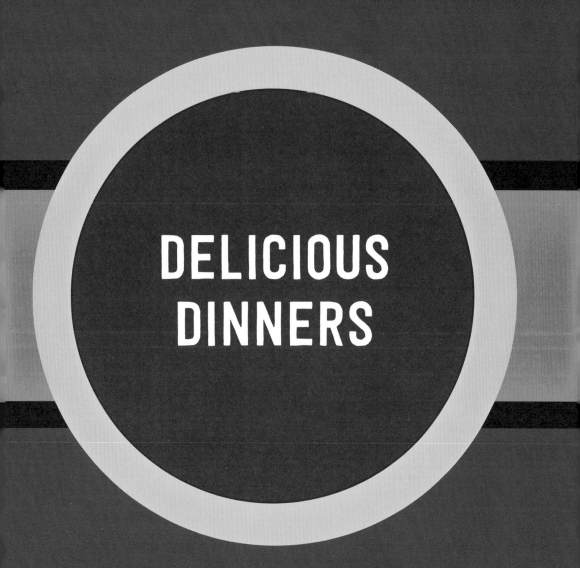

DELICIOUS DINNERS

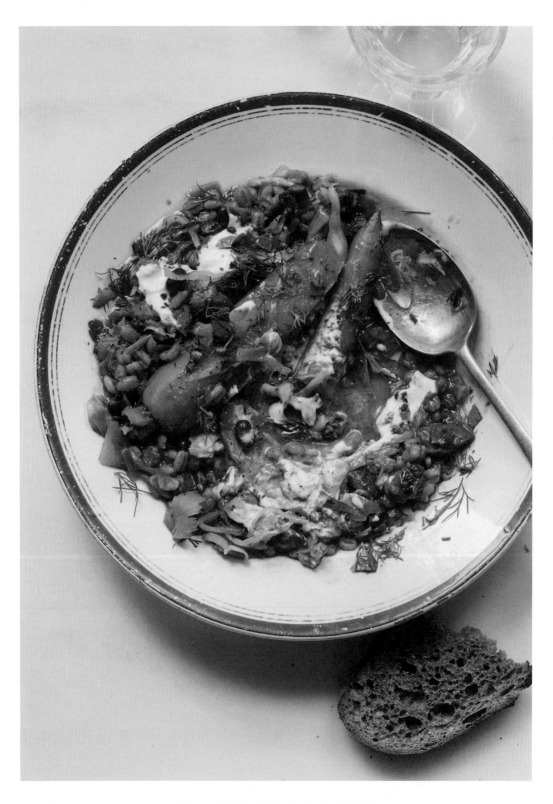

BARLEY, BLACK BEAN & MUSHROOM STEW

15g (½oz) dried porcini mushrooms

3 tablespoons olive oil, plus extra to serve

225g (8oz) mixed fresh mushrooms, cleaned, trimmed and torn into equal-sized chunks

1 onion, finely chopped

1 small leek, trimmed, quartered and well washed, then sliced

3 garlic cloves, chopped

1 bay leaf

8 small whole carrots

1 celery stick, finely diced

200g (7oz) pearl barley, well rinsed and drained

1½ teaspoons smoked paprika

½ teaspoon ground cumin

½ teaspoon turmeric

1 teaspoon tomato purée

1 small glass (125m/¼fl oz) red wine

1½ teaspoons brown miso paste

900ml (1½ pints) just-boiled water

400g (14oz) can black beans, or 200g (7oz) black beans from a jar

100g (3½oz) Vadasz Garlic & Dill Sauerkraut or homemade Sauerkraut With Garlic & Dill (see page 26}

1 teaspoon honey or maple syrup

salt and pepper

TO SERVE

4 tablespoons soured cream or dairy-free alternative

1 big pinch of chopped flat leaf parsley or dill

1 pinch of pul biber/Aleppo chilli flakes or Turkish chilli flakes

toasted bread

This is a recipe that combines traditional Hungarian flavours with a nod to a classic Shabbat cholent, or *sólet* as it's known in Hungary. Purists might frown at this veggie take on such a traditionally meaty dish – it's clearly nothing like an original cholent, which is made with smoked goose or brisket, but the sauerkraut adds depth and acidity, and creates a lovely wholesome bowl of stew.

Put the dried porcini in a small bowl and pour over about 100ml (3½fl oz) just-boiled water to cover, then set aside to soak for about 10 minutes.

While the mushrooms are soaking, heat the olive oil in a large flameproof casserole dish or saucepan over a medium heat. Add the mixed fresh mushrooms, season well with salt and pepper and cook for 6–8 minutes, until starting to brown.

Lift out the soaked porcini mushrooms, reserving the soaking liquid, and roughly chop. Add to the pan, followed by the onion, leek, garlic and bay leaf. Cook for another 3–5 minute, until the onion and leek have softened but not browned.

Add the carrots, celery and barley and cook, stirring, for 1–2 minutes.

Reduce the heat, add all the spices and the tomato purée and stir well for 1 minute, until the barley is all coated and the pan dry but not catching.

Add the wine and bubble away for a minute or so, scraping the bottom of the pan with a wooden spoon to loosen any of the caramelized bits.

Stir in the miso paste and the porcini soaking liquid, pouring it in through a sieve to catch any grit, and add the measured just-boiled water. Season with salt and pepper (but remember the miso is salty), then cover the pan and simmer gently for about 30 minutes, until the barley is tender but not too soft – al dente is good!

Add the black beans and their liquid, the sauerkraut and honey or maple syrup and warm through for 5–10 minutes. Taste and add more salt and pepper if needed.

Ladle into big bowls, topped with a generous swirl of soured cream, the chopped parsley or dill, a good glug of extra olive oil and the chilli flakes. Serve with toasted bread to scoop and dip.

TUNA, MACKEREL & PICKLED FENNEL BUCATINI

I used to throw a glass of white wine into this sauce and reduce it in the pan to enrich the result, but since I've had so much brine in my life, I now add pickle brine instead, resulting in the same desired acidity, plus some sweetness and a big bold layer of pickle flavour too, which I really love! This dish exemplifies how the use of pickle brine can add value to your day-to-day cooking. Try it with some Vadasz Red Onion Fresh Pickles or homemade Pickled Red Onions (see page 38) as an alternative to the fennel. Using both tuna and mackerel gives the sauce a deeper fish flavour, but feel free to use whatever you have in your cupboard. Make sure it's the best canned fish in oil — preferably olive oil. Spread any remaining sauce over a crusty slice of bread, crostini or pizza base for a very satisfying snack or starter.

2 tablespoons olive oil, plus extra to serve

1 onion, thinly sliced

2 garlic cloves, chopped

1 tablespoon Pickled Fennel with Lemon (see page 44), plus extra to serve, and 2 tablespoons of the brine

about 145g (5oz) canned tuna in oil, including the oil

125g (4½oz) canned mackerel fillets in oil, including the oil

400g (14oz) cherry tomatoes, halved

1 handful of pitted green olives, squeezed and broken up or crumbled as they leave your hand

1 tablespoon small capers, drained

2 pinches of chilli flakes

350g (12oz) bucatini or other long pasta

1 big handful of basil leaves

salt and pepper

TO GARNISH

Parmesan cheese, for grating

1 small handful of flat leaf parsley, chopped

Fill a large pan with salted water, cover with a lid and bring to the boil.

While the water is heating up, heat the olive oil in a large frying pan over a medium heat. Add the onion, garlic and pickled fennel and sweat gently, stirring frequently, for about 5 minutes, until soft.

Pour in the brine, stirring and shaking to loosen the onion and fennel from the bottom of the pan, then add all the remaining ingredients, except the pasta and basil leaves, and season with salt and pepper. Mix together gently — you want to retain some texture of the fish — and bring them to a simmer. Cover the pan and cook nice and gently for about 15 minutes.

While the sauce is simmering gently, cook the pasta according to the packet instructions until al dente.

When the pasta is cooked, taste the sauce for salt and pepper and stir through the basil leaves. Using tongs or similar, lift the pasta from the boiling water directly into your pan of tuna and mackerel sauce; as you do so, the starchy water clinging to the pasta will help add body to the sauce. Mix the pasta through the sauce with a fork and a spoon until it's well combined.

Serve in your favourite pasta bowls and top with a scattering of the extra pickled fennel, a generous grating of Parmesan, the chopped parsley and some bold swirls of olive oil.

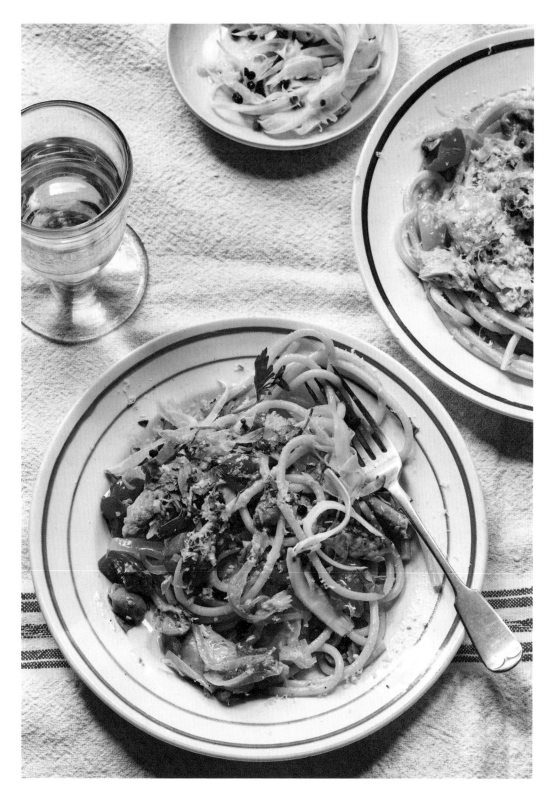

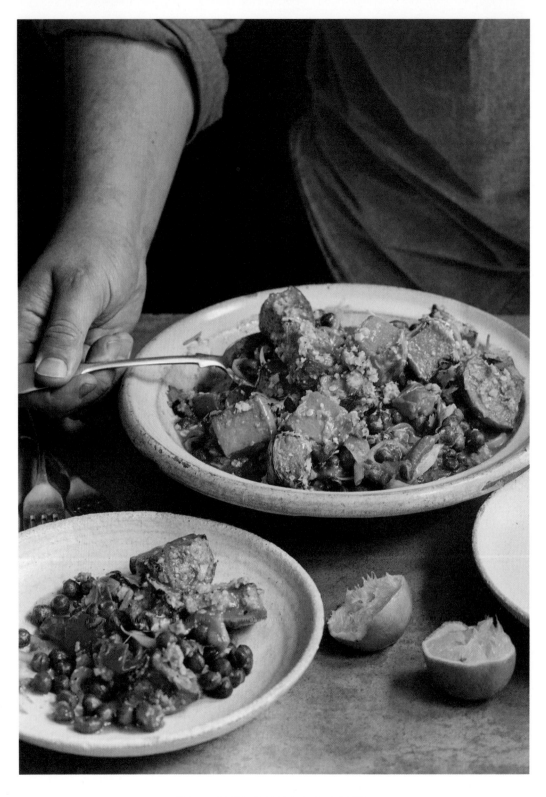

COCONUT SQUASH CURRY WITH BRAISED CARLIN PEAS

1 squash (butternut or red kuri), about 700–800g (1lb 9oz–1lb 12oz), scrubbed, halved lengthways, deseeded and sliced into large chunks about 3cm (1¼ inches) thick

olive oil, for roasting

2 tablespoons extra virgin olive oil, plus extra to serve

1 onion, finely diced or sliced

2 garlic cloves, crushed

3 tomatoes, chopped

1 bay leaf

2½ teaspoons garam masala

700g (1lb 9oz) jar Carlin peas, including their liquid

salt and pepper

FOR THE CURRY PASTE

40g (1½oz) fresh root ginger, scrubbed and chopped

5 garlic cloves, chopped

1 red chilli, chopped

4 tablespoons Vadasz Pineapple & Turmeric Sauerkraut or homemade Curried Kraut (see page 27)

2 tablespoons coconut chips

1 tablespoon vegetable oil, plus extra for cooking

1 big pinch each of salt and pepper

TO SERVE

1 lime wedge, for squeezing over

small handful of coriander, chopped

chilli sauce (optional)

The firm yet giving nature of roasted squash means it's able to absorb any flavour you throw at it, in this case a curry paste featuring pineapple and turmeric sauerkraut and coconut chips, resulting in a sweet, spicy dry curry. I've matched that with a braise of Carlin peas, which really are worth seeking out, though if you can't get them, red kidney beans also work well.

Preheat your oven to 220°C/200°C fan (425°F), Gas Mark 7. Put the squash on a baking tray, drizzle with olive oil and toss to coat, then spread out in a single layer and roast for about 30–35 minutes, until soft and slightly charred.

While the squash is roasting, prepare the curry paste. Add all the ingredients to a mini food processor or a blender and blend to a coarse but well-formed paste — you'll want to retain some texture, so don't overblend. Set aside.

Heat the extra virgin olive oil in a wide deep frying pan over a medium heat. Add the onion and sweat for about 2 minutes. Add the garlic, tomatoes, bay leaf and garam masala and cook, stirring, for 1–2 minutes before adding the Carlin peas or red kidney beans and their liquid. Season to taste with salt and pepper, cover the pan and simmer gently for 5–10 minutes. Turn off the heat and leave to rest with the lid on.

Once the squash is cooked, place a heavy-based deep frying pan over a high heat and, when hot, add the curry paste along with a drop of vegetable oil and stir-fry for 1–2 minutes. Add the squash and cook, continuing to stir and shaking the pan frequently, for about 5–6 minutes until charred but not burned.

To serve, spoon the peas or beans into large wide bowls, then pile up the curried squash pieces. Pour over a generous swirl of extra virgin olive oil, add a squeeze of juice from the lime wedge and scatter over the chopped coriander. Some really good chilli sauce won't go amiss either.

CRISPY CAULIFLOWER KIMCHEESE

My mum used to make me something she named 'crispy cauliflower surprise'.
The surprise was, in fact, a can of baked beans and mini sausages buried
beneath the cauliflower and béchamel – oh, the glamour of the 1970s!
Nevertheless, the way the bean juice (as we called it) bled into the white
sauce and added its distinctive sweet-savoury tomato tang was really lovely.
The addition of kimchi in this dish delivers a similarly delectable experience.

1 large cauliflower

1 large leek, trimmed, rinsed and cut into 6 pieces

2 tablespoons olive oil

½ tablespoon gochujang (Korean red chilli paste

2–3 tablespoons Vadasz Kimchi or homemade Kimchi (see page 24), plus 1 tablespoon of the kimchi brine

salt and pepper

FOR THE BÉCHAMEL SAUCE

800ml (1⅓ pints) whole milk

25g (1oz) butter

drop of olive oil

2 tablespoons plain flour

2 teaspoons English mustard

1 bay leaf

1 pinch of ground cloves

½ teaspoon ground or freshly grated nutmeg

½ tablespoon gochujang/Korean red chilli paste

2 handfuls of grated mature Cheddar cheese, plus 2 handfuls for topping

Preheat your oven to 220°C/200°C fan (425°F), Gas Mark 7.

Heat a deep ovenproof frying pan over a medium heat while you prepare
the cauliflower. Trim the stem base and remove the tough outer leaves
to leave the inner leaves intact. Hold the cauliflower, stem end down, on
a chopping board and cut into slices 2cm (¾ inch) thick – you should
get about 4, plus some florets.

Put the cauliflower steaks and florets in a large bowl along with the leek and
1 tablespoon of the olive oil. Mix the gochujang with the extra tablespoon of
the kimchi brine, add to the cauliflower and mix together gently.

Add the remaining 1 tablespoon of olive oil to the hot pan. Season the
cauliflower steaks and florets with salt and pepper, add to the pan – in
batches if necessary – and sear for about 5 minutes on each side, until
nice and brown and a little charred too, turning once or twice. Transfer
to a dish and cover snugly with foil to let the residual heat continue the
cooking while you prepare the béchamel sauce.

Pour half the milk into a large measuring jug and set aside. Add the
butter and a drop of olive oil to the empty pan over a gentle heat and,
when melted, add the flour and stir well to combine and make a roux.
Cook, stirring continuously, for about 2 minutes – avoid colouring the
roux too much.

Tip the roux into the milk in the jug and use a stick blender to carefully
blitz until combined and smooth. Pour it into the pan and add the
remaining milk along with the mustard, bay leaf, spices, gochujang
and salt and pepper. Mix well, then bring to a very gentle simmer and
cook, stirring continuously, until the sauce is thick and creamy. Add the
cheese and whisk vigorously to combine.

Take the pan off the heat and add the cauliflower and leeks, pushing
them down into the sauce until you have semi-submerged veggie buoys.
Top generously with the kimchi and the extra cheese and slide the pan
into the oven for 20 minutes, or until the kimcheese topping is crisp
and browned and the béchamel beneath is bubbling like volcanic lava.
Serve immediately.

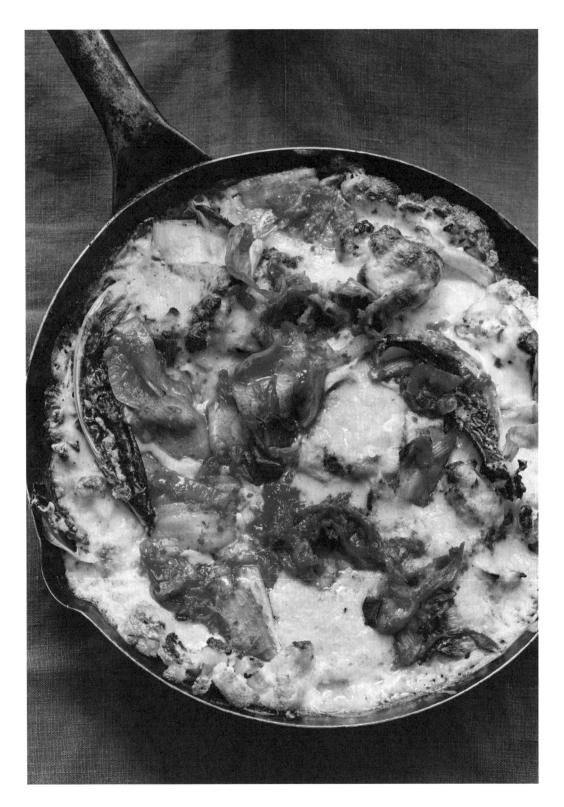

BRAISED BEANS WITH CHEESE & PICKLE

I love beans, and I really love black beans. This simple recipe is almost always served in my house with jalapeño relish, cheese and often pickled red onions too, and I also love them with simply buttered corn kernels and rice. I use these beans in the Tortilla Salad on page 110, but try using them in the Breakfast Quesadilla on page 56 or add to the pan, before the eggs, for a more substantial version of the tortilla chips, salsa and eggs on page 64.

2 tablespoons olive oil

1 onion, finely diced

2 garlic cloves, chopped

1 tomato, chopped

I bay leaf

1 big pinch of dried oregano (Mexican if possible) or 1 sprig of fresh oregano

2 x 400g (14oz) cans black or pinto beans

salt and pepper

TO SERVE

feta cheese, crumbled

Vadasz Red Onion Pickles or homemade Pickled Red Onions (see page 38)

1 handful of coriander, chopped

Vadasz Jalapeño Relish or homemade Jalapeño Relish (see page 49)

Heat the olive oil in a medium-sized saucepan over a medium heat. Add the onion and garlic and sweat for 3 minutes. Then add the tomato, season with salt and pepper and cook for another 3 minutes.

Stir in the bay leaf and oregano, then add the beans and their liquid. Mix well, bring to a gentle simmer and cook, covered loosely with a lid, for 20 minutes.

Take the pan off the heat and, using the back of a wooden spoon, mash some of the beans against the side of the pan until the mixture thickens. Cover the pan until you are ready to serve them – they will continue to thicken.

Serve the beans topped with the crumbled feta, pickled red onions, chopped coriander and jalapeño relish.

SHEPHERD'S KIMCHI PIE

I love a good pie, especially a potato-topped one. I think I could do a whole recipe book just on shepherd's pies, from a global perspective. So to me, the idea of making a keema-inspired lamb curry and topping it with spiced, fresh coriander-flecked creamy mash, or a Hungarian-style version with paprika, sauerkraut and soured cream, isn't odd at all, and I have done so often, with delicious results. But this version has to be one of my favourites, where kimchi's spicy, funky acidity, along with buttery, creamy mash, perfectly balances the lamb's lovely rich, full-fat flavour.

800g (1lb 12oz) minced lamb

1 onion, sliced

2 carrots, diced

½ celery stick, diced

1 bay leaf

1 tablespoon tomato purée

1 tablespoon gochujang (Korean red chilli paste)

100g (3½oz) Vadasz Kimchi or homemade Kimchi (see page 24), plus 2 tablespoons of the brine

salt and pepper

FOR THE MASHED POTATOES

1kg (2lb 4oz) floury potatoes

160g (5¾oz) Vadasz Kimchi or homemade Kimchi (see page 24)

40g (1½oz) butter

TO SERVE

cooked fine green beans

Vadasz Kimchi or homemade Kimchi (see page 24)

For the mash, peel the potatoes, then halve or quarter them if necessary so that they are roughly the same size. Rinse to remove the excess starch, drain and put in a large pan. Cover with cold salted water, bring to the boil and cook for about 15 minutes, until soft enough to break when prodded with a fork but still retain some texture. Drain well, reserving 350ml (12fl oz) of the cooking water, and let them steam-dry in the colander for a couple of minutes.

While the potatoes are boiling, heat a heavy-based ovenproof frying pan over a high heat. Season your minced lamb well with salt and pepper, add to the hot pan and fry for 10–12 minutes, until well browned and crusty, getting as much flavour as you can from the lamb – you might need to drain some of the fat off at this stage.

Add the onion, carrots, celery, bay leaf, tomato purée and gochujang and cook, stirring, for a minute. Pour the brine and reserved potato cooking water into the pan and stir rapidly, loosening the lamb from the bottom of the pan. Add the kimchi, then cover the pan, reduce the heat and simmer for 30 minutes or so.

While the lamb is simmering gently, mash the cooked potatoes, adding the kimchi, butter and some salt and pepper. Once mashed, whip together vigorously until smooth and creamy. Preheat the oven to 220°C/200°C fan (425°F), Gas Mark 7.

After the lamb has simmered for 30 minutes or so, top with the mashed potatoes, placing big spoonfuls in a circle until you've covered it all. Smooth out using a spatula, then use a fork to create some texture on the surface. Bake for 15–20 minutes, until the mashed potato topping is well browned. Serve immediately with fine green beans and a big spoonful of raw kimchi.

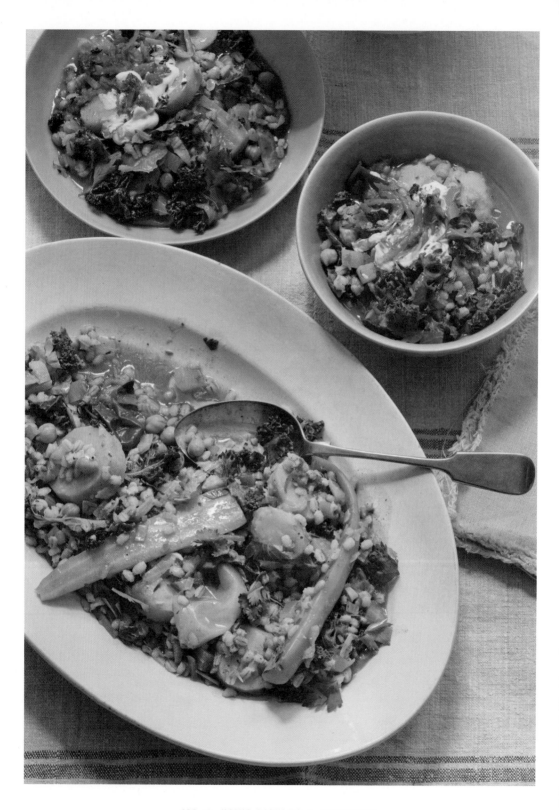

PARSNIP, DAIKON & BARLEY TAGINE WITH KIMCHI

2 tablespoons olive oil, plus extra to serve

1 onion, finely diced

3 garlic cloves, finely chopped

2 large parsnips (about 250g/8oz), sliced into large rounds, or 6 baby parsnips, left whole

4 carrots (about 225g/8oz), halved lengthways, or 8 small carrots, left whole

250g (9oz) daikon, cut into large dice

1 small piece of celery, finely sliced

1 teaspoon paprika

1 teaspoon ground ginger

1 teaspoon ground cumin

½ teaspoon turmeric

1 bay leaf

200g (7oz) pearl barley, well washed and drained

2 large or 4 medium tomatoes, quartered

240g (8½oz) canned, drained chickpeas

200g (7oz) Vadasz Kimchi or homemade Kimchi (see page 24), plus extra to serve

1 litre (1¾ pints) water

2 big handfuls of chopped kale

salt and pepper

TO SERVE

1 big handful of chopped coriander or flat leaf parsley

1 big spoonful of thick natural yogurt (optional)

½ teaspoon cumin seeds, toasted (optional)

Early on in my career as a chef toiling away in kitchens across London, I was fortunate to work with many colleagues from Morocco and Algeria, and became immersed in and a little obsessed with the now-familiar flavours of North African cuisine: cumin, preserved lemons, merguez and roast peppers. I particularly loved the *chorba* and *harira* soups, which were often prepared for staff meals or during Ramadan for *iftar*, the fast-breaking evening meal. But it was the deeply savoury, spicy tagine that I enjoyed most and that I still cook regularly. Often served with couscous, here I've used barley as the grain to pull it all together. The vegetables are cut large or left whole to retain flavour, and instead of preserved lemons, kimchi serves us well yet again to add the requisite acidity along with a kick of chilli.

Heat the olive oil in a large flameproof casserole dish or saucepan over a medium-high heat. Add the onion and sweat for 1–2 minutes, stirring continuously. Add the garlic, all the veg and a big pinch of salt and pepper and stir well.

Cover the pan, reduce the heat and cook for 2–3 minutes. Remove the lid, stir in the spices and bay leaf and keep stirring for another minute or so, then add the barley, tomatoes, chickpeas and kimchi along with the measured water. Mix well and taste for salt and pepper.

Replace the lid and bring to the boil, then reduce the heat and simmer nice and gently for 40–45 minutes, until the barley is tender but retains some bite and the vegetables are well cooked.

Stir through the kale and taste for salt and pepper, then turn the heat off and let it rest with the lid on for 5–10 minutes.

Serve in big bowls with a swirl of olive oil, the extra kimchi, the chopped coriander or parsley, and perhaps a big spoonful of thick natural yogurt and some toasted cumin seeds if you like.

KIMCHI PESTO PASTA

I've always enjoyed playing around with pasta and sauces, so here I've reimagined pesto with kimchi and Thai basil. Unless you're a purist, anything goes — even Marmite, hey Nigella! Try spreading the pesto on to crostini for mezze or into a baguette for a very special garlic bread. If not using straight away, put in a lidded container with more olive oil on top to preserve it and store in the fridge, where it will last for a week.

100g (3½oz) pine nuts

3 big tablespoons of Vadasz Kimchi or homemade Kimchi (see page 24)

40g (1½oz) Thai basil (or use regular basil if you can't find it)

1–2 garlic cloves, peeled

4 tablespoons good extra virgin olive oil

1 lime, halved, for squeezing

40g (1½oz) Pecorino Romano or Parmesan cheese, grated

600g (1lb 5oz) pasta of your choice, cooked

salt and pepper

Toast the pine nuts in a large, dry frying pan for 1–2 minutes, until light golden, then tip on to a plate to cool slightly.

Put the toasted pine nuts, kimchi, basil, garlic, 2 tablespoons of the olive oil and a squeeze of lime juice in a mini food processor or a blender and pulse until well blended but retaining some texture.

Using a spatula, scrape the mixture into a bowl and stir through the cheese and remaining olive oil. Season with salt, pepper and a squeeze more lime juice to taste.

Stir into your favourite cooked pasta with a little of the pasta water, then serve with extra grated cheese.

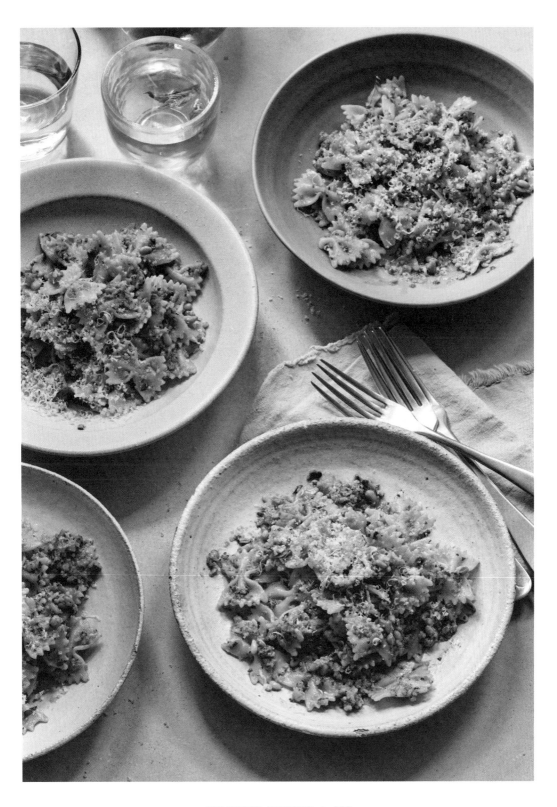

CURRY KRAUT CHICKEN CURRY WITH GREEN APPLE CHUTNEY

Who doesn't love a chicken curry? This is a nod to a classic butter chicken, with the warm, earthy flavours of Vadasz Pineapple & Turmeric Sauerkraut, or your homemade equivalent, doing most of the spice work and demonstrating it's amazing versatility!

2 tablespoons vegetable oil

6 boneless, skinless chicken thighs

2 onions, halved and sliced

3 garlic cloves, chopped

2 large tomatoes, quartered

3 heaped tablespoons Vadasz Pineapple & Turmeric Sauerkraut or homemade Curried Kraut (see page 27)

60g (2¼oz) cashew nuts

400ml (14fl oz) can coconut milk

a knob of butter

1 large baking potato, peeled and cut into 2cm (¾-inch) cubes

1 cinnamon stick

1 or 2 bay leaves

1 hot red chilli, halved lengthways (optional)

salt and pepper

TO SERVE

Green Apple Chilli Chutney (see page 43)

1 handful of coriander leaves

cooked brown or white basmati rice

Heat 1 tablespoon of the vegetable oil in a large, heavy-based frying pan over a medium heat. Season the chicken thighs with salt and pepper, add to the pan and fry gently for 10 minutes, turning halfway through, until nicely browned all over. Transfer to a plate and set aside.

Add the remaining 1 tablespoon oil to the pan, followed by the onions and garlic and cook for 2 minutes, stirring to loosen the chicken residue from the base. Add the tomatoes, sauerkraut and cashews with a pinch more salt and pepper, and cook for another 1–2 minutes, until you get the wonderful aromas of curry beginning to fill your kitchen.

Stir in the coconut milk, then cover the pan, bring the contents back up to a simmer and simmer for 5–6 minutes.

Add the butter to the pan, then take off the heat. Tilt the pan slightly and use a stick blender to blitz the mixture until it's thicker and saucier, but don't overdo it — it's always nice to have some textural components too.

Return the chicken thighs to the pan with all their juices and the potato. Drop in the cinnamon stick, bay leaves and chilli, if using, slide the pan back on to a medium heat and stir well. Cover and simmer gently for about 50 minutes or until the chicken is really tender — you might need to add a drop of water if the curry is too thick, but it shouldn't need much if you keep the pan well covered and the heat low.

Serve topped with a big dollop of the apple chilli chutney, some coriander leaves and brown or white basmati rice on the side.

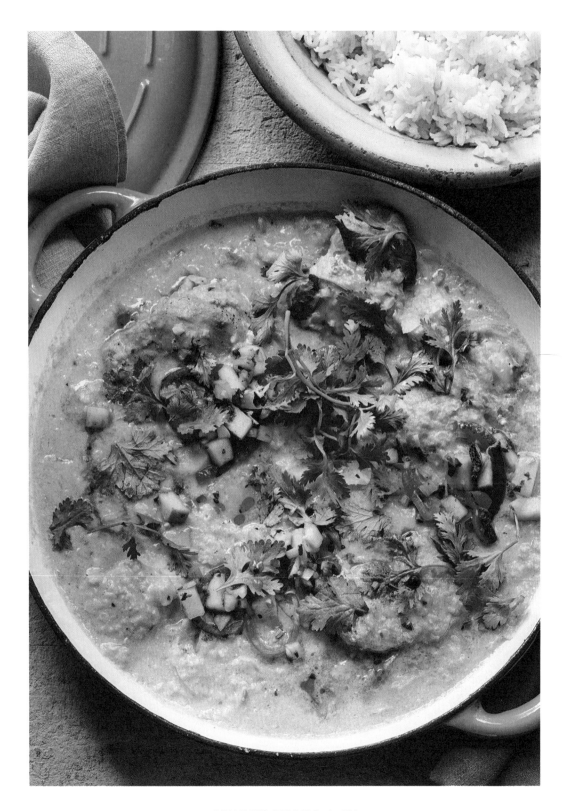

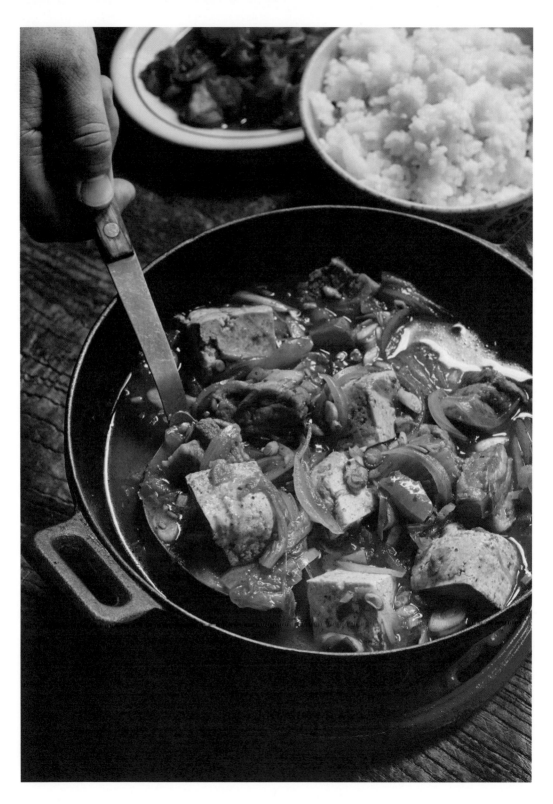

KIMCHI STEW

Kimchi *jjigae* is one of those dishes that really makes the most out of kimchi and, just as paprika is synonymous with *gulyás* (goulash) in representing Hungarian cuisine, this most popular Korean dish promotes kimchi at its heart. Delicious and deeply satisfying umami flavours will resonate long after your bowl is finished. I've made my version, inspired by those I've eaten here in London, with pork belly, but for vegans and vegetarians, meat can easily be omitted, along with the fish sauce, and replaced by a miso-based stock with just the tofu.

300g (10½oz) pork belly, sliced into strips 2cm (¾ inch) wide, top layer of skin removed

200g (7oz) Vadasz Kimchi or homemade Kimchi (see page 24), plus a little extra to serve, and 2 tablespoons of the brine

1 small or ½ large leek, trimmed, rinsed and cut across into large slices

1 onion, halved and thickly sliced

2 spring onions, sliced, reserving some to garnish

1 tablespoon maple syrup

1 tablespoon gochujang (Korean red chilli paste)

2 teaspoons gochugaru (Korean red chilli flakes)

1 teaspoon sesame oil

1 teaspoon salt

1 tablespoon fish sauce

1 tablespoon soy sauce

500ml (18fl oz) just-boiled water

225g (8oz) pressed firm or silky tofu, sliced into 4cm (1½-inch) squares or big bite-sized chunks

cooked short-grain rice, to serve

Put the pork into a large, wide saucepan and cover with all the other ingredients, except the tofu, pouring the just-boiled water over last.

Cover the pan, bring to a rapid simmer and cook for 15 minutes.

Remove the lid and add the tofu, then replace the lid and cook for 5–6 minutes, until warmed through.

Serve in bowls on a bed of cooked short-grain rice, garnished with the reserved spring onions and a little more kimchi.

KIMCHI SPECIAL FRIED RICE

Why is special fried rice special? Well, because it's special. It's a busy bowl of rice often scattered with various meats, fish, peas and eggs, and like all great rice dishes, it's a meal in itself. It's also special because it's often made from leftovers, so there's an opportunity to raid the fridge and use stuff up. My version has some extra ingredients to elevate it to ultra-special status, namely kimchi, gochujang and sesame, plus I use short-grain rice, which makes for a stickier result than long grain. You can add any cold cooked meats, or you can go plant-based, swapping the eggs for tofu and going heavy on the vegetables, cutting anything raw finely. Get all your ingredients prepped and ready to cook, as this all comes together really quickly. You have been warned!

1 tablespoon vegetable oil

4 eggs, beaten

250g (9oz) cooked chicken or pork, finely diced

150–175g (5½–6oz) raw peeled prawns

½ bunch of spring onions, cut into thick slices at an angle

1 thumb-sized piece of fresh root ginger, scrubbed and cut into very thin strips

2 garlic cloves, chopped

3 tablespoons soy sauce

3 tablespoons sesame oil

1 tablespoon gochujang/Korean red chilli paste

400g (14oz) short-grain rice, cooked – leave in a wide dish to cool down before you use it (yesterday's cooked chilled rice is ideal)

100g (3½oz) Vadasz Kimchi or homemade Kimchi (see page 24), plus extra to serve

150g (5½oz) frozen peas

TO SERVE

large handful of chopped coriander

sesame seeds, for sprinkling

hot sauce or chilli oil

Heat a wok or large frying pan over a high heat and add the vegetable oil, rotating and tilting the pan to cover the surface well. When smoking hot, add the beaten eggs, again rotating the pan so that they cover the oiled base and the lower side of the pan. At the same time, using a metal or wooden spatula, scrape the eggs back and forth to break them up as they cook rapidly — they should take less than 30 seconds.

Add the meat, prawns, spring onions, ginger and garlic, shaking and moving the ingredients in the pan continuously. Then add the soy sauce, sesame oil and gochujang, stirring and shaking vigorously until they are all thoroughly mixed.

Stir in the rice, kimchi and peas, and continue to stir and scrape, moving and mixing the rice with the other ingredients, for about 5 minutes, or until it's piping hot.

To serve, pile up on plates, adding the extra kimchi, chopped coriander, a sprinkle of sesame seeds and a dash of your favourite hot sauce or chilli oil.

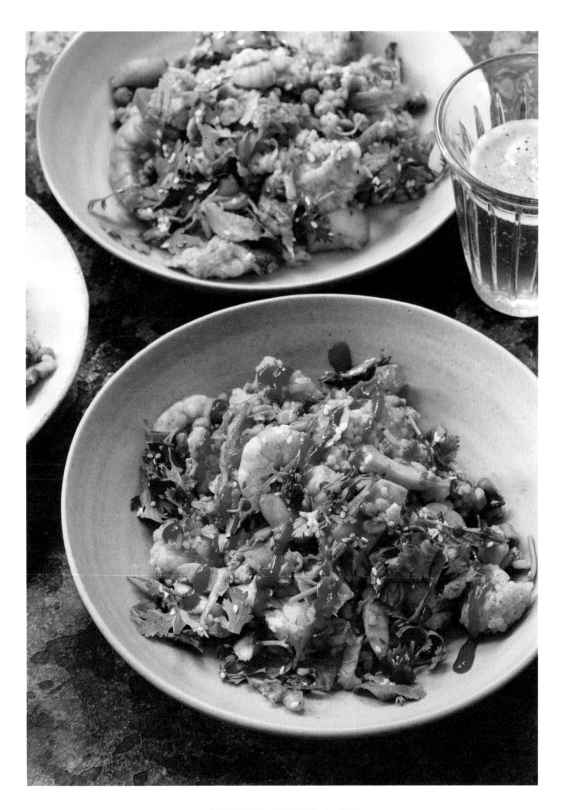

SMALL PLATES & DRINKS

TEMPURA FRIED PICKLES

I remember eating 'frickles' at a restaurant a few years back and I wasn't impressed, as the batter was too heavy and greasy, so I was determined to create a lighter, better version. I've made them here with a mixture of cucumber pickle slices, whole pickled okra and slices of chillies en escabeche, but you can also make little patties with a mix of sauerkraut and kimchi (Vadasz or see pages 24 and 25 for recipes) by scooping portions in a tablespoon and squeezing out the brine, then dredging, still in the spoon, through the batter before frying. These are great as a starter, snack or side accompanied by this quick homemade dip.

8–10 slices of Vadasz Garlic & Dill Pickles or Quick Cucumber Pickle (see page 41)

3–6 whole Pickled Okra (see page 39)

1 handful of Vadasz Red Onion Pickles or homemade Pickled Red Onions (see page 38)

8–12 whole jalapeños or large mixed chillies (about 2 x 100g/3½oz packs), cut into 1cm (½ inch) slices

vegetable oil, for shallow-frying

FOR THE HONEY MUSTARD DIP

3 tablespoons mayonnaise

2 teaspoons Dijon mustard

2 teaspoons Fermented Honey with Garlic & Chilli (see page 33) or regular clear honey

salt and pepper

FOR THE BATTER

85g (3oz) cornflour

40g (1½oz) plain flour

1 teaspoon baking powder

200ml (7fl oz) ice-cold sparkling water

First make the dip. Put all the ingredients in a small serving bowl and mix well. Set aside

Drain all the pickles well and pat dry with kitchen paper.

Pour 1cm (½ inch) vegetable oil into a large saucepan and heat to 170°C (340°F). If you don't have a thermometer, drop a small cube of bread into the hot oil, and when it turns golden in 30 seconds, the oil is ready.

While the oil is heating up, make the batter. Add the dry ingredients to a large mixing bowl with some salt and pepper and mix together, then whisk in the sparkling water thoroughly until you have a smooth batter.

When the oil has reached the required temperature, use chopsticks or a fork to submerge the pickles in the batter, turning them over to coat well. When they are all coated, gently but quickly, using tongs if you like, cast them into the hot oil – in 2 or more batches, if using a smaller pan – and fry for 1½–2 minutes on each side, until golden and crisp. Transfer to a plate lined with kitchen paper to absorb the excess oil. Serve immediately piled up around the dip.

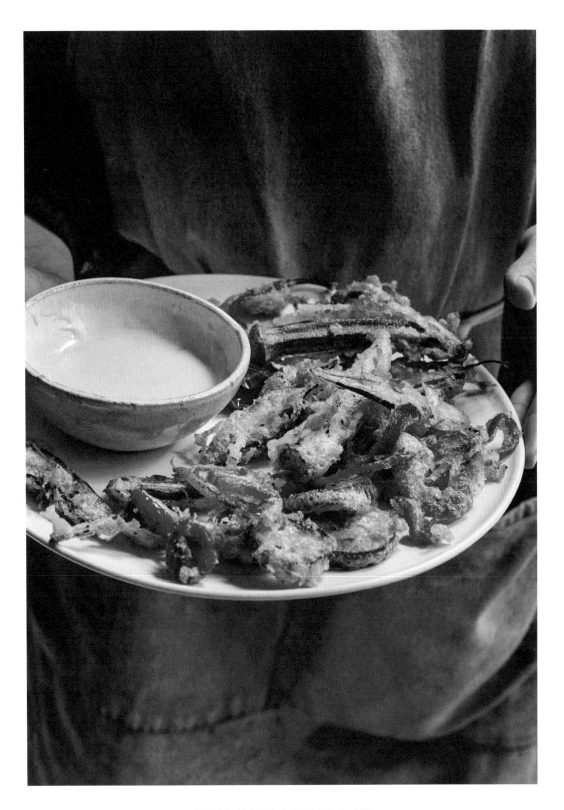

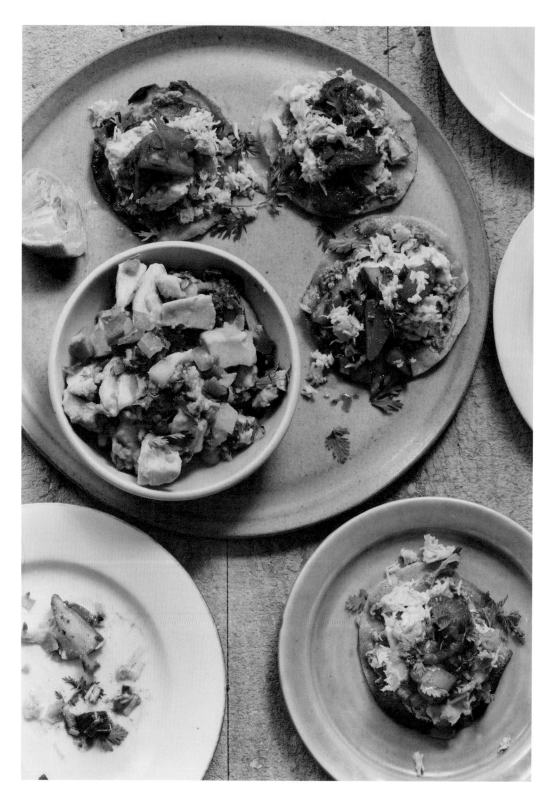

CRAB & AVOCADO TOSTADAS

This classic canapé is well worth embellishing with a little pickle love.
I've used the sweet, tart and fiery Pineapple, Strawberry & Cucumber
Salsa, which complements it so well, to create a tantalizing sip
of the coast in summer for you and your guests.
If you want to make this as a starter or snack instead of a canapé,
simply use two 15cm (6-Inch) corn tortillas, shallow-fried until crisp
and then rested and cooled, before topping.

1 avocado

½ tablespoon mayonnaise

juice of ¼ lime

15–20 round plain corn chips

85g (3oz) mixed white and brown
crabmeat

Pineapple, Strawberry & Cucumber Salsa
(see page 36)

salt and pepper

coriander leaves, to garnish

Slice the avocado in half lengthways and remove the stone. Using a
dessertspoon, scoop the flesh into a small bowl. Chop and mash the
avocado with the spoon just a little bit while you mix in the mayo,
lime juice and a good pinch of salt and pepper.

Lay out the corn chips on your work surface. To each add 1 teaspoon
avocado mixture, 1 big pinch of crabmeat and 1–2 teaspoons salsa,
then top with 1 or 2 coriander leaves to garnish. Arrange on a large
plate and serve.

AVOCADO & JALAPEÑO SALSA

Years ago, when working in a Tex-Mex restaurant in London, I recall a harsh, concentrated lime juice product used mainly for margaritas but that proclaimed 'makes great guacamole' on the packaging, and we did indeed mix it with the avocados. I'm very glad to say that we've since progressed to using fresh limes, and there are now countless good Mexican restaurants and food businesses in London — even the Tex-Mex ones have improved. I usually keep it simple when making guacamole, just using ripe avocados, seasoning and a squeeze of lime, but I call this rendition a salsa, as the jalapeño relish punches through the soft avocado with its acidity, heat and some sweetness, and underlying is the gorgeous hum of coriander. As well as enjoying with corn chips as a dip, try it it in addition to the tomato and red pepper salsa in Tortilla Chips with Fresh Salsa & Eggs on page 64 or alongside the Cheese & Pickle Breakfast Quesadillas on page 56.

3 ripe Hass avocados

juice of 1 lime, plus an extra squeeze if storing

2 tablespoons Vadasz Jalapeño Relish or homemade Jalapeño Relish (see page 49), well drained

1 big handful of coriander, roughly chopped

2 big pinches of salt

1 big pinch of pepper

Slice the avocados in half lengthways and remove the stones, reserving one if not using the salsa straight away. Using a dessertspoon, scoop the avocado flesh into a bowl. Then slice the avocado with the edge of the spoon until you have roughly chopped it — but keep it chunky.

Add the other ingredients and stir well to combine. Taste for salt, adding more if needed.

If not using straight away, transfer the salsa to a food storage container, drop the reserved stone in the centre and add a squeeze more of lime before putting on the lid — this will preserve it and prevent discoloration until you want to use it. It will keep in the fridge for 1–2 days.

KIMCHI HUMMUS WITH MINT & CORIANDER OIL

Pairing silky smooth hummus with spicy, herb-heavy olive oil for dipping is such a good way to kick off a big dinner or to enjoy as a lunchtime treat or snack, and the addition of kimchi really elevates the hummus to another level. Try using butter beans or even black beans instead of the classic chickpeas.

3 garlic cloves, roughly crushed

60g (2¼oz) Vadasz Kimchi or homemade Kimchi (see page 24), plus extra to serve

250g (9oz) canned or jarred chickpeas, plus 85g (3oz) for serving, drained

40g (1½ oz) tahini

juice of ½ lemon

1 big pinch each of salt and pepper

2 tablespoons extra virgin olive oil

FOR THE HERB OIL

1 handful of mint

1 handful of coriander

1 pinch each of salt and pepper

4 tablespoons extra virgin olive oil

TO SERVE

1 spring onion, very finely sliced

hunks of warm baguette or pitta breads

First make the herb oil. Put the herbs and salt and pepper in a food processor or blender and, as you blend them, drizzle in the olive oil until well combined. Transfer the oil to a small jug or bowl and set aside.

Rinse out the bowl of the food processor or blender, add all the ingredients for the hummus, except the oil, and blend well. Remove the lid and use a flexible spatula to scrape down the sides now and then to ensure all the ingredients hit the blades. Then with the machine running, drizzle in the oil until the mixture has emulsified and you have a smooth, creamy blend. Keep blending and add more oil to increase the smoothness if you like. Taste for texture and seasoning. Transfer the hummus to a wide, shallow bowl or plate.

Place a tablespoon at the centre of the hummus and push down with the back of it while you rotate your bowl or plate to create a shallow bath in the centre. Load your extra kimchi along with the chickpeas and spring onions into the well, and drizzle over the herb oil. Serve with hunks of just-out-of-the-oven crusty baguette or pitta breads.

KIMCHI PRAWN COCKTAIL

Call me old-fashioned, but I am very partial to a prawn cocktail, and back in the days when this old favourite was a starter option on most menus in restaurants up and down the land, I, along with most of my family, would invariably order it, wishing there had been just a little bit more of it (and the accompanying brown bread and butter too). Most contemporary versions are ubercool, served on ice, the cocktail sauce tomato-heavy with no mayo, tasting more like a bloody Mary than a Marie Rose. My sauce looks like a Marie Rose but more orangey, and tastes sweet enough, but there's a tartness from the kimchi and lemon, plus it's a little spicier and a touch more rustic than the classic. Serve it in tall, wide cocktail glasses for best effect.

300g (10½oz) large cooked peeled prawns, patted dry with kitchen paper

1 Little Gem lettuce

1 tablespoon sesame seeds

1 lemon, quartered

4 slices of quality wholemeal bread, generously buttered

FOR THE MARIE ROSE SAUCE

3 tablespoons mayonnaise

1 garlic clove, finely chopped

1 heaped tablespoon Vadasz Kimchi or homemade Kimchi (see page 24), finely chopped

1 teaspoon gochujang/Korean red chilli paste

1 teaspoon maple syrup

grated zest and juice of ¼ lemon

1 pinch each of salt and pepper

First make the Marie Rose sauce. Put all the ingredients in a small bowl and mix well.

Roughly chop half the prawns into smaller pieces, put in a separate bowl and cover with 4 tablespoons of the sauce. Add the remaining whole prawns to another bowl along with 1–2 tablespoons of the sauce or just enough to coat them. You should have some sauce left for topping the cocktail.

Finely shred one half of the lettuce and slice the other half lengthways into 4 long quarters.

Toast the sesame seeds in a dry frying pan over a high heat, shaking the pan continuously, for about 2 minutes, until they are lightly coloured.

To serve, divide the shredded lettuce between your cocktail glasses and insert the lettuce quarters on one side. Divide the chopped, sauced prawns between the glasses and hang the whole prawns around the rim of the glasses.

Finish off by dolloping any remaining sauce on top, sprinkling with the toasted sesame seeds and balancing a lemon quarter on the side of each glass. Serve with the buttered bread.

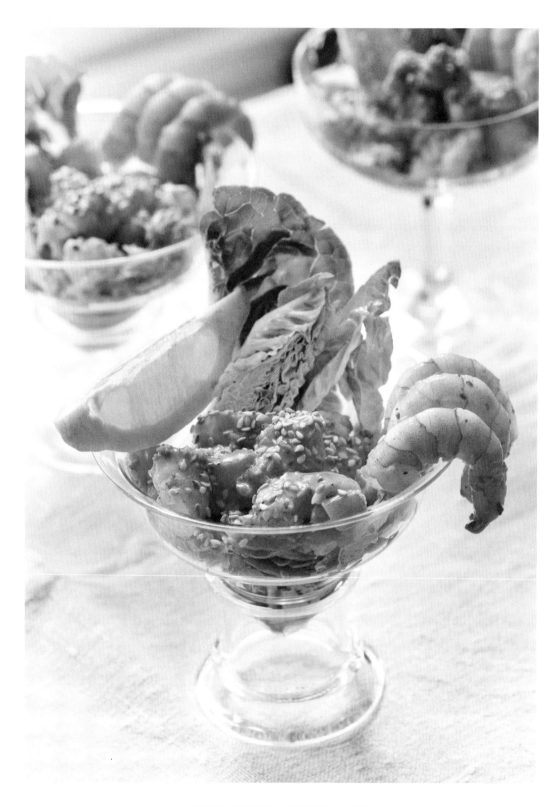

KIMCHI PRAWN & SESAME TOAST CRUMPETS WITH KIMCHI MISO SYRUP

I well remember the excitement and joy of eating out in Chinatown as a child. One of my favourite things to eat was sesame prawn toast, the crispy fried bread topped with a thick, juicy, bouncy layer of minced prawns sprinkled with sesame seeds. Quick and easy to replicate at home, I've taken the opportunity to get creative by adding kimchi to the prawn mix and kimchi brine to the dipping sauce. And I've used crumpets instead of bread to absorb all the buttery goodness.

165g (5¾oz) uncooked peeled prawns, chilled

2 tablespoons Vadasz Kimchi or homemade Kimchi (see page 24), chilled, plus extra to serve

1 egg, white and yolk separated, yolk beaten

1 tablespoon soy sauce

1 teaspoon sesame oil

4 crumpets

25g (1oz) butter

½ tablespoon vegetable oil

4 tablespoons sesame seeds

1 big pinch of finely chopped spring onions, to serve

FOR THE KIMCHI MISO SYRUP

½ teaspoon brown miso paste

3 tablespoons of the kimchi brine

1 tablespoon maple or golden syrup

1 teaspoon sesame oil

grated zest and juice of ½ lemon

First make the kimchi miso syrup. Add the miso paste to a small ramekin or serving bowl and thin with the kimchi brine. Then add the other ingredients and mix well.

Put the prawns, kimchi, the egg white, soy sauce and sesame oil in a food processor or blender and blend to a paste but still retaining a little bit of texture from the prawns.

Heat a large, heavy-based frying pan over a low heat. While the pan is heating up, use a spatula to generously smear the prawn paste over the top of each crumpet, pushing down firmly as you load it on to ensure it's well covered. Then use the spatula to smooth the paste out around the edges of your crumpets — you want a good thick layer on each one.

Once the pan is hot, add the butter and vegetable oil. Brush each prawn-topped crumpet, including the sides, with the beaten egg yolk and sprinkle generously with the sesame seeds.

Carefully slide each crumpet into the pan, bottom side down, and fry gently for 1–2 minutes, until browned. Carefully turn them over and fry the prawn-topped side for 2–3 minutes, or until browned and firm/ bouncy to the touch.

Serve the crumpets whole or cut in half with the kimchi miso syrup, a sprinkle of spring onions and some extra kimchi.

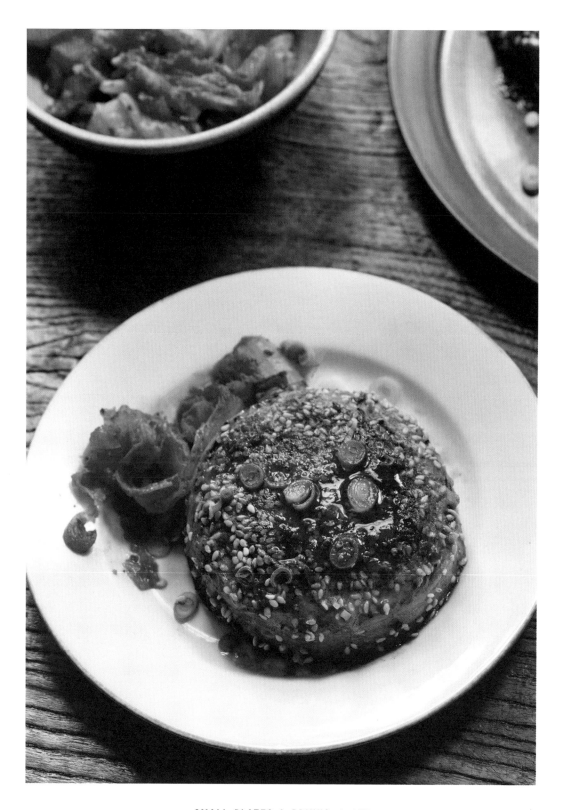

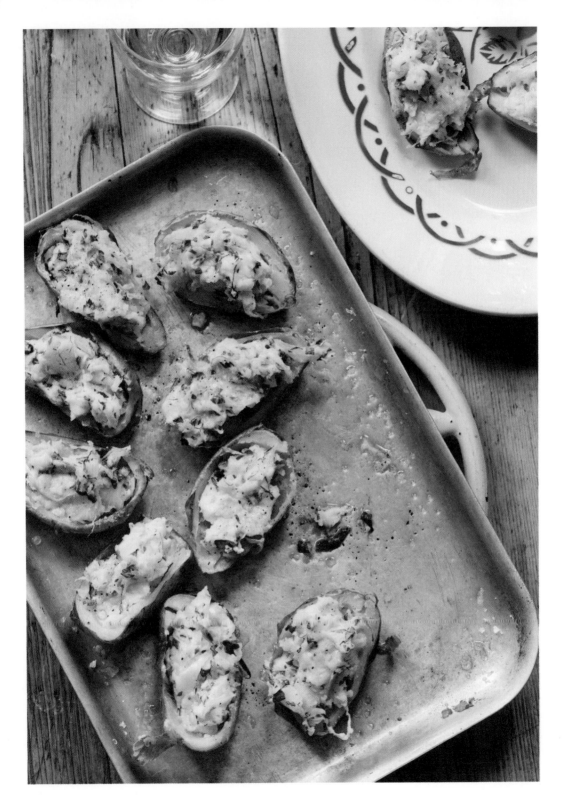

SAUERKRAUT & CHEESE-STUFFED BAKED POTATOES

When I'm away working, it seems baked potatoes get eaten a lot in our house, and according to my son, while not complaining, the familiar filling options of baked beans, cheese and tuna mayo get a bit boring after a while. So as a solution, I've taken a tip from the Netherlands, where sauerkraut is combined with creamy mashed potatoes (and often bacon too) to great effect, and used a similar approach for stuffing baked potatoes. But I've raised the game even further with the addition of cream cheese (or feta). Result: one happy boy!

vegetable oil

4 large floury potatoes (such as Maris Piper), scrubbed

100g (3½oz) Vadasz Garlic & Dill Sauerkraut or homemade Sauerkraut with Garlic & Dill (see page 26)

1 heaped tablespoon cream cheese or crumbled feta cheese

1 tablespoon soured cream

1 handful of flat-leaf parsley, chopped

25g (1oz) butter, plus extra to serve

salt and pepper

salad, to serve

Preheat your oven to 220°C/200°C fan (425°F), Gas Mark 7, or an air fryer to 180°C (350°F).

Drizzle your potatoes with vegetable oil and sprinkle with a little salt, then bake in the oven for 50 minutes, or cook in the air fryer for 45 minutes.

While the potatoes are cooking, put the sauerkraut, cream cheese or feta, soured cream, parsley and a good pinch each of salt and pepper in a large bowl and mix together well.

To check the potatoes are done, put on a clean oven glove or use a clean tea towel to squeeze them gently to see if they are soft inside, then transfer to a work surface or chopping board. Cut the potatoes in half lengthways and carefully scoop the flesh into your cheese mixture, leaving the skins intact. Add the butter and, using a flexible spatula, mix or whip well until creamy but still slightly textured. Taste and add more salt and pepper if needed.

Holding each skin in turn in one hand, use the spatula to fill with your potato mixture, overfilling them as much as you can.

Return the stuffed potatoes to the oven or air fryer and heat them through for 5 minutes, or until they colour slightly. Serve with a little more butter to melt on top of each one and a lovely fresh salad. No baked beans or tuna!

CHICKEN WINGS WITH FERMENTED HONEY SAUCE

Trying these for the first time with my eldest son at a chicken wing festival in London, I recall struggling with their overwhelming chilli heat and gasping for air. But that wasn't enough to put me off, and captivated by their crispy, gochujang beauty, I soon polished them off, their skeletal remains, a pile of orange-stained napkins and my sticky fingers evidence of my newfound obsession. My version is hot, yes, but not crazy hot, and all the other elements are here to get you hooked. Try swapping out the chicken for cauliflower florets and losing the fish sauce for a veggie alternative.

3 tablespoons cornflour

vegetable oil – spray works well here

9–12 chicken wings

salt and pepper

FOR THE SAUCE

3 tablespoons Fermented Honey with Garlic & Chilli (see page 33)

1 tablespoon gochujang/Korean red chilli paste

1 tablespoon soy sauce

1 tablespoon tomato ketchup

1 tablespoon apple cider vinegar

½ tablespoon sesame oil

½ tablespoon fish sauce

TO SERVE

a good handful of Vadasz Kimchi or homemade Kimchi (see page 24)

3 finely sliced spring onions

finely sliced cucumber, cut into matchsticks

1 tablespoon sesame seeds

Preheat your oven to 240°C/220°C fan (475°F), Gas Mark 9, or an air fryer to 200°C (400°F).

Put the cornflour in a freezer bag and season it with some salt and pepper.

Spray or brush the chicken wings lightly with vegetable oil, then add them to the bag and seal. Shake until the wings are well coated with the seasoned flour.

Spread the wings out on a large baking tray and bake for 25 minutes, or put them on the base of the air fryer and cook for 15 minutes.

While the wings are cooking, make the sauce. Put all the ingredients in a mixing bowl large enough to accommodate the wings and mix well until you have a smooth, thick and glossy sauce.

After 25 minutes in the oven or 15 minutes in the air fryer, turn the wings over and cook for another 5 minutes, or until cooked through. Remove from the oven or air fryer and let them rest for 5 minutes.

Drop your rested wings into the bowl of sauce and stir thoroughly to fully coat them. Using tongs, arrange them on serving plates along with a generous spoonful of kimchi, the spring onions, cucumber and sesame seeds. Serve with plenty of kitchen paper.

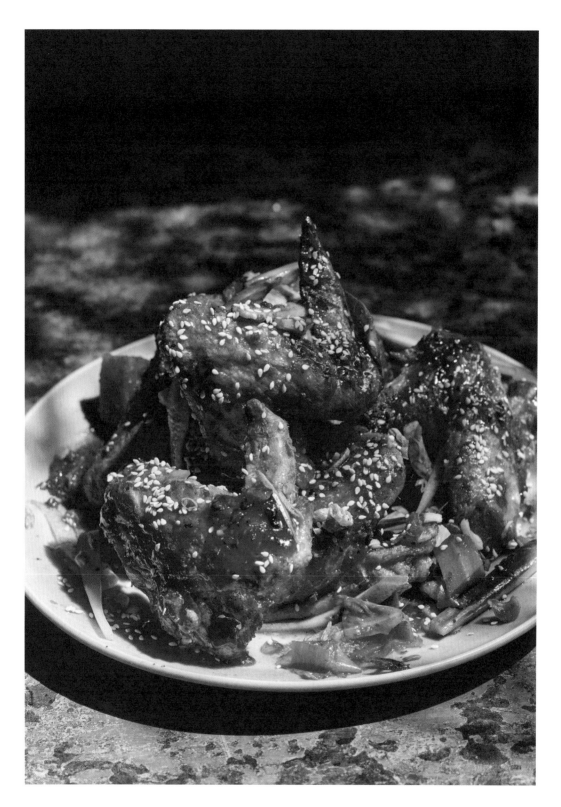

DIMA'S VODKA COCKTAILS

Making time to enjoy a cocktail or two with friends is the perfect aperitif to set you up for the meal you are about to eat, and Dima's Vodka really hits the spot. I first met Dima in 2022, when he generously provided his Dima's Vodka for a Cook For Ukraine charity event we hosted at Mission Kitchen, London. It was a very special day that brought together some amazing chefs who prepared the most delicious dinner for our guests, as well as Dima's Vodka cocktails using Vadasz pickles and brine. It was so good, we are still raving about them to this day.

In Ukraine, just as in Hungary where my family are from, pickles and the brine they bathe in are often paired with drinks — in Ukraine it's generally vodka all the way. Dima runs a very successful vodka business, supplying some of the UK's best bars, restaurants and retailers. The following recipes have been specially developed by Dima — the perfect match for savoury, tangy pickles and brine.

Enjoy, and please raise your glasses for the traditional Ukrainian toast:
Budmo!

SERVES 1

50ml (2fl oz) Dima's Vodka

3 dashes Worcestershire sauce

1 dash Tabasco sauce

½ teaspoon horseradish sauce

25ml (1fl oz) brine from Vadasz Super-Beet Kimchi or homemade Beetroot Kimchi (see page 25), plus 1 teaspoon of the beetroot kimchi to serve

tomato juice, to taste

ice

1 sprig of dill, to garnish

BEETROOT MARY

Put the vodka, Worcestershire sauce, Tabasco, horseradish and beetroot kimchi brine in a highball glass.

Top up with tomato juice to your taste, then add ice and stir to combine.

Garnish with the sprig of dill and serve with the beetroot kimchi on the side to eat just before drinking.

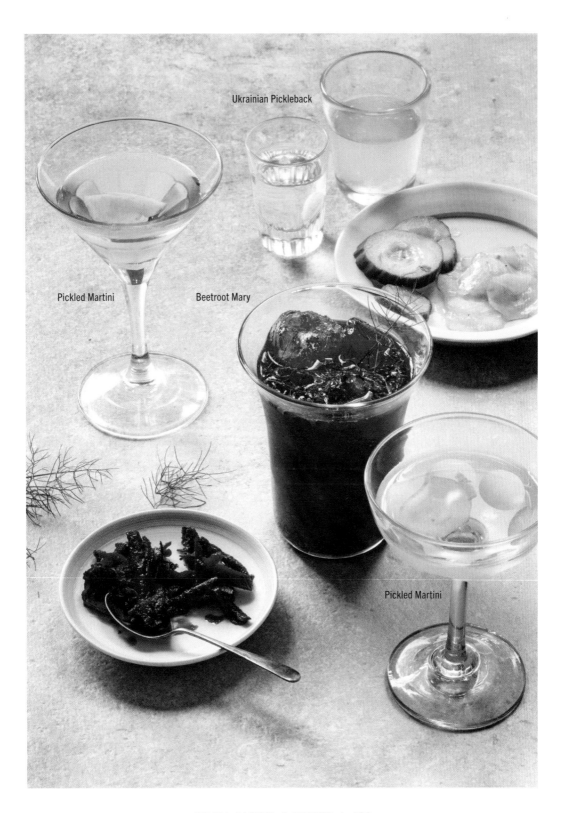

Ukrainian Pickleback

Pickled Martini

Beetroot Mary

Pickled Martini

PICKLED MARTINI

ice

70ml (2¼fl oz) Dima's Vodka

1 tablespoon brine from Vadasz Garlic & Dill Pickles or homemade Quick Cucumber Pickle (see page 41), plus 1 slice of the cucumber pickle to serve

25ml (1fl oz) white vermouth

Put some ice in a highball glass, add the vodka, pickle brine and white vermouth and stir to combine. Alternatively, add the ice and ingredients to a cocktail shaker and shake to combine and chill.

Strain into a chilled martini glass and add the slice of pickled cucumber.

UKRAINIAN PICKLEBACK

50ml (2fl oz) Dima's Vodka

50ml (2fl oz) brine from Vadasz Garlic & Dill Pickles or homemade Quick Cucumber Pickle (see page 41)

Drink the shot of vodka, then follow immediately with the shot of pickle brine!

KIMCHI MOCKTAILS

You don't necessarily need alcohol to enjoy the benefits that pickled and fermented brine bring to the party, when it comes to cocktails. The bright colours and funky depth of flavour you get with these two mocktails will really hit the spot and hopefully get you creating many more.

SERVES 1

ice

160ml (5½fl oz) pressed pineapple juice

4 teaspoons brine from Vadasz Kimchi or homemade Kimchi (see page 24), plus 1 pinch of the kimchi to serve

50ml (2fl oz) freshly squeezed orange juice

2 teaspoons raspberry cordial

1 big slice of orange

KIMCHI SUNRISE

Put some ice in a highball glass and pour over the pineapple juice.

Slowly add the kimchi brine and the orange juice, followed by the raspberry cordial.

Serve with a big slice of orange, the pinch of kimchi and a cocktail spoon to stir.

SERVES 1

ice

2 teaspoons brine from Vadasz Super-Beet Kimchi or homemade Beetroot Kimchi (see page 25), plus 1 pinch of the beetroot kimchi to serve

2 teaspoons blackcurrant cordial

1 lime, halved

150ml (5fl oz/¼ pint) tonic water

IF YOU CAN'T BEET IT, DRINK IT

Put some ice in a highball glass, pour over the beetroot kimchi brine and blackcurrant cordial and squeeze over the juice from one lime half. Stir well to combine.

Top up with the tonic water, then add the remaining lime half, squeezing it as you do so, and the pinch of beetroot kimchi to garnish.

REFERENCES & FURTHER READING

An, S-Y, Lee, M S, Jeon J Y, Ha E S, Kim T H, Yoon J Y, Ok C-O, Lee H-K, Hwang W-S, Choe S J, et al., 'Beneficial effects of fresh and fermented kimchi in prediabetic individuals', *Annals of Nutrition and Metabolism*, 2013; 63: 111–19

Bousquet J, Anto J M, Czarlewski W, Haahtela T, Fonseca S C, Iaccarino G, Blain H, Vidal A, Sheikh A, Akdis C A, et al., 'Cabbage and fermented vegetables: From death rate heterogeneity in countries to candidates for mitigation strategies of severe COVID-19', *Allergy: European Journal of Allergy and Clinical Immunology*, 2021; 76: 735–50

Cai W, Tang F, Wang Y, Zhang Z, Xue Y, Zhao X, Guo Z and Shan C, 'Bacterial diversity and flavor profile of Zha-Chili, a traditional fermented food in China', *Food Research International*, 2021; 141: 110112

Choi I H, Noh J S, Han J-S, Kim H J, Han E-S and Song Y O, 'Kimchi, a fermented vegetable, improves serum lipid profiles in healthy young adults: randomized clinical trial', *Journal of Medicinal Food*, 2013; 16: 223–9

Chung H G, Min Y W, Lee C, Hong S N, Won J Y, Jang J A, Kim C-H and Chang D K, 'Effects of novel probiotics in a murine model of irritable bowel syndrome', *Korean Journal of Gastroenterology*, 2020; 75: 141–6

Graudal N and Jürgens G, 'Conflicting evidence on health effects associated with salt reduction calls for a redesign of the salt dietary guidelines', *Progress in Cardiovascular Diseases*, 2018; 61: 20–6

Han Y-M, Kang E A, Park J M, Oh J Y, Lee D Y, Choi S H and Hahm K B, 'Dietary intake of fermented kimchi prevented colitis-associated cancer', *Journal of Clinical Biochemistry and Nutrition*, 2020; 67: 263–73

Han Y-M, Park J-M, Jeong M, Yoo J-H, Kim W-H, Shin S-P, Ko W-J and Hahm K-B, 'Dietary, non-microbial intervention to prevent *Helicobacter pylori*-associated gastric diseases', *Annals of Translational Medicine*, 2015; 3: 122

He G-Q, Liu T-J, Sadiq F A, Gu J-S and Zhang G-H, 'Insights into the microbial diversity and community dynamics of Chinese traditional fermented foods from using high-throughput sequencing approaches', *Journal of Zhejiang University Science B*, 2017; 18: 289–302

Henry C J, 'Functional foods', *European Journal of Clinical Nutrition*, 2010; 64: 657–9

Kim H-Y and Park K-Y, 'Clinical trials of kimchi intakes on the regulation of metabolic parameters and colon health in healthy Korean young adults', *Journal of Functional Foods*, 2018; 47: 325–33

Lee S Y, Sekhon S S, Ko J H, Kim H C, Kim S Y, Won K, Ahn J-Y, Lee K and Kim Y-H, 'Lactic acid bacteria isolated from kimchi to evaluate anti-obesity effect in high fat diet-induced obese mice', *Toxicology and Environmental Health Sciences*, 2018; 10: 11–16

Liu L, Du P, Zhang G, Mao X, Zhao Y, Wang J, Duan C, Li C and Li X, 'Residual nitrite and biogenic amines of traditional northeast sauerkraut in China', *International Journal of Food Properties*, 2017; 20: 2448–55

Lorn D, Nguyen T-K-C, Ho P-H, Tan R, Licandro H and Waché Y, 'Screening of lactic acid bacteria for their potential use as aromatic starters in fermented vegetables', *International Journal of Food Microbiology*, 2021; 350: 109242

Mallappa R H, Balasubramaniam C, Nataraj B H, Ramesh C, Kadyan S, Pradhan D, Muniyappa S K and Grover S, 'Microbial diversity and functionality of traditional fermented milk products of India: Current scenario and future perspectives', *International Dairy Journal*, 2021; 114: 104941

Nielsen E S, Garnås E, Jensen K J, Hansen L H, Olsen P S, Ritz C, Krych L and Nielsen D S, 'Lacto-fermented sauerkraut improves symptoms in IBS patients independent of product pasteurisation – a pilot study', *Food & Function*, 2018; 9: 5323–35

Orgeron R P, II, Corbin A and Scott B, 'Sauerkraut: A Probiotic Super-food', *Functional Foods in Health and Disease*, 2016; 6: 536—43

Park J M, Han Y M, Oh J Y, Lee D Y, Choi S H, Kim S J and Hahm K B, 'Fermented kimchi rejuvenated precancerous atrophic gastritis via mitigating *Helicobacter pylori*-associated endoplasmic reticulum and oxidative stress', *Journal of Clinical Biochemistry and Nutrition*, 2021; 69: 158—70

Park J M, Lee W H, Seo H, Oh J Y, Lee D Y, Kim S J and Hahm K B, 'Microbiota changes with fermented kimchi contributed to either the amelioration or rejuvenation of *Helicobacter pylori*-associated chronic atrophic gastritis', *Journal of Clinical Biochemistry and Nutrition*, 2021; 69: 98—110

Park S-E, Kwon S J, Cho K-M, Seo S-H, Kim E-J, Unno T, Bok S-H, Park D-H and Son H-S, 'Intervention with kimchi microbial community ameliorates obesity by regulating gut microbiota', *Journal of Microbiology*, 2020; 58: 859—67

Peñas E, Martínez-Villaluenga C and Frías J, 'Sauerkraut: Production, composition, and health benefits' in Frias J, Martinez- Villaluenga C and Peñas E, eds, *Fermented Foods in Health and Disease Prevention*, Academic Press, London, UK, 2016; pp. 557—70

Peñas E, Martínez-Villaluenga C, Frías J, Sánchez-Martínez M J, Pérez-Corona M T, Madrid Y, Cámara C and Vidal-Valverde C, 'Se improves indole glucosinolate hydrolysis products content, Se-methylselenocysteine content, antioxidant capacity and potential anti-inflammatory properties of sauerkraut', *Food Chemistry*, 2012; 132: 907—14

Raak C, Ostermann T, Boehm K and Molsberger F, 'Regular consumption of sauerkraut and its effect on human health: A bibliometric analysis', *Global Advances in Health and Medicine*, 2014; 3: 12—18

Sawicka H, 'Glucosinolates as natural plant substances – structural and application aspects: A review', *Journal of Cell and Tissue Research*, 2020; 20: 6919—28

Seong G, Lee S, Min Y W, Jang Y S, Kim H S, Kim E-J, Park S-Y, Kim C-H and Chang D K, 'Effect of heat-killed *Lactobacillus casei* DKGF7 on a rat model of irritable bowel syndrome', *Nutrients*, 2021; 13: 568

Septembre-Malaterre A, Remize F and Poucheret P, 'Fruits and vegetables, as a source of nutritional compounds and phytochemicals: Changes in bioactive compounds during lactic fermentation', *Food Research International*, 2018; 104: 86—99

Sivamaruthi B S, Kesika P, Prasanth M I and Chaiyasut C, 'A mini review on antidiabetic properties of fermented foods', *Nutrients*, 2018; 10: 1973

Stiemsma L T, Nakamura R E, Nguyen J G and Michels K B, 'Does consumption of fermented foods modify the human gut microbiota?', *Journal of Nutrition*, 2020; 150: 1680—92

Varzakas T, Zakynthinos G, Proestos C and Radwanska M, 'Fermented vegetables' in Yildiz F and Wiliey R, eds, *Minimally Processed Refrigerated Fruits and Vegetables*, Springer Science, New York, USA, 2017; pp. 537—84

INDEX

Bold pagination indicates main pickle recipes